EASY
GASTRIC SLEEVE
BARIATRIC
COOKBOOK

Easy GASTRIC SLEEVE

BARIATRIC COOKBOOK

100 Recipes for Healing and Sustainable Weight Loss

MARINA SAVELYEVA, RD, CNSC

PHOTOGRAPHY BY
ANDREW PURCELL

ROCKRIDGE
PRESS

Interior and Cover Designer: John Calmeyer
Art Producer: Tom Hood
Editor: Rachelle Cihonski
Production Editor: Matthew Burnett

Photography ©2020 Andrew Purcell. Food styling by Carrie Purcell. Author photo courtesy of Irina Pop, IrinkArt-Photo
Cover: Egg and Avocado Toast, page 95

ISBN: Print 978-1-64739-779-1 | eBook 978-1-64739-465-3
R0

THIS BOOK IS DEDICATED

to all gastric sleeve patients as well as the bariatric surgeons, nurses, dietitians, therapists, and other clinicians who help patients achieve their goals and support them in embracing a healthy lifestyle.

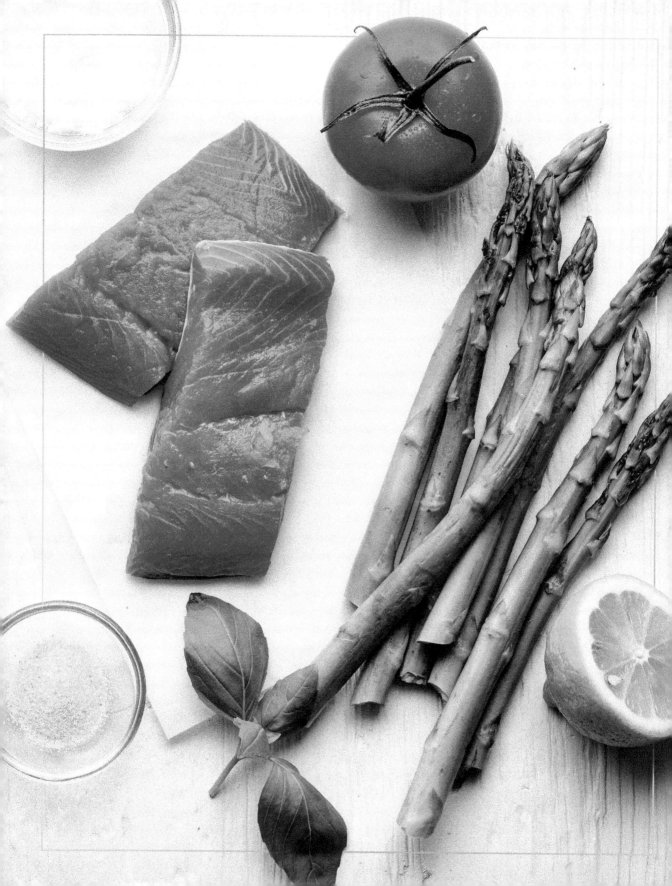

CONTENTS

INTRODUCTION

When I was growing up in Russia, my mom taught me how to cook from scratch at an early age. We never ate out in restaurants, and fast food was not an option. I realize now how great it was to eat homemade meals cooked with fresh ingredients. As I grew older, I loved experimenting with new recipes and came to understand how important nutrition is for health and well-being. This led to my pursuit of a degree in food science.

After college, I immigrated to the United States, where I completed my bachelor of science degree in food science and nutrition. Then I finished one year of supervised practice, passed the national exam, and became a Registered Dietitian Nutritionist.

My first job was working for a bariatric surgeon in Palm Springs, California. Early on, I learned how important it is for patients to have great follow-up care, education, and support. I created educational brochures for patients as well as a variety of nutrition classes, grocery lists, and grocery store tours. The surgeon and I also followed up closely with patients after surgery.

For the past 15 years I've worked with a few different bariatric surgeons, attended conferences and support groups, and seen many gastric sleeve patients for counseling. Many of these patients who were admitted to the hospital shared their nutrition stories with me.

Sometimes, patients are blamed for not following instructions, possibly resulting in weight gain or complications after surgery. But I've found it's not always the patient's fault. Many people do not receive great follow-up care and education, and many struggle with understanding what to eat and what not to eat. I've also noticed a lot of information—sometimes conflicting—given by medical professionals or online.

If you've picked up this book and are contemplating having (or have already had) gastric sleeve surgery, I can assure you that you've made the right decision to have the surgery. Successful patients follow up with their surgeon and a dietitian, attend support groups, and continuously learn about their own well-being.

The goal of this book is to provide education about how to eat after surgery and to make the process as easy as possible.

I want you to enjoy the process of healing and losing weight after gastric sleeve surgery, to learn healthy habits, and to enjoy the foods you eat. Before we dive into the details, however, I want to give you a few tips based on my experience working with and hearing from bariatric patients.

» *First, don't compare yourself, your progress, or your weight loss with other patients.* After gastric sleeve surgery, your stomach size will depend on the surgeon's discretion. Every surgeon is different, but the standard amount of stomach left after surgery is between one-third and one-fourth its original size. The new stomach usually accommodates anywhere from two to six ounces of food. Some patients may end up with a smaller stomach than others. Therefore, you should not compare yourself to other patients— even with the same surgeon. Every patient is unique and has a different medical condition, stomach size, and lifestyle. Your unique journey is yours alone.

» *Second, don't rely solely on health care professionals or your family for support. Rely, for the most part, on yourself.* I've seen patients who aren't interested in learning how to cook for themselves and instead expect their families or hired help to prepare meals for them. However, no one else can eat for you. It is not only about the food you eat; it's also about how you eat it. You are the one who needs to develop new life skills, such as eating slowly and chewing food properly. Although they are a great support system and source of encouragement, your surgeon, dietitian, partner, and family cannot help you all the time. It is important to learn all the information, take notes, and take care of yourself.

» *Lastly, it is okay to have some bad days or get off track. Life happens.* When setbacks happen, try to get back on track as fast as you can. Be compassionate toward yourself and don't criticize yourself: Negativity will only postpone your progress and success.

My wish for you is that you have a healthy life and thrive after gastric sleeve surgery. Take care of your body. It is your home—otherwise, where will you live?

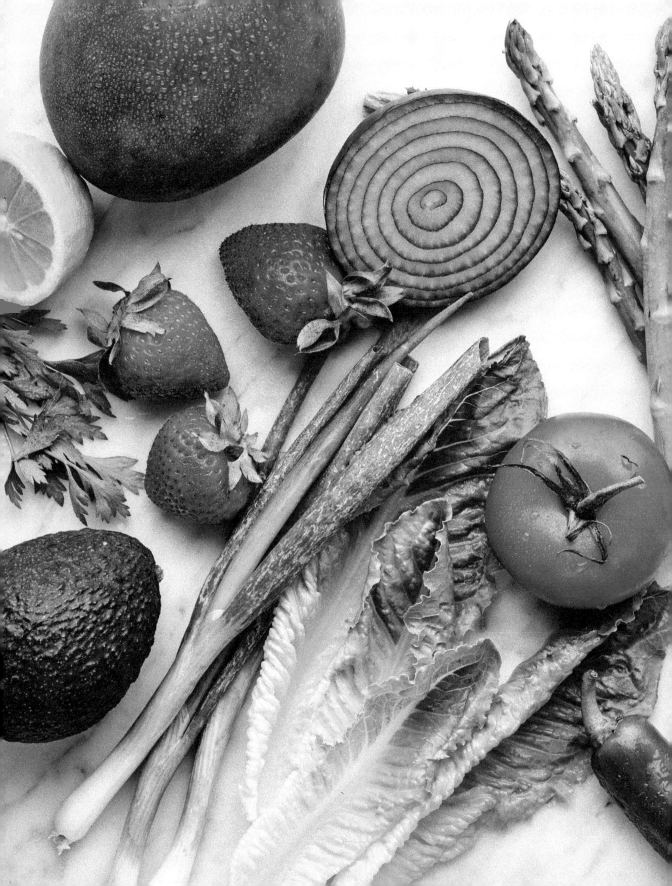

PART ONE

THE SLEEVE SOLUTION

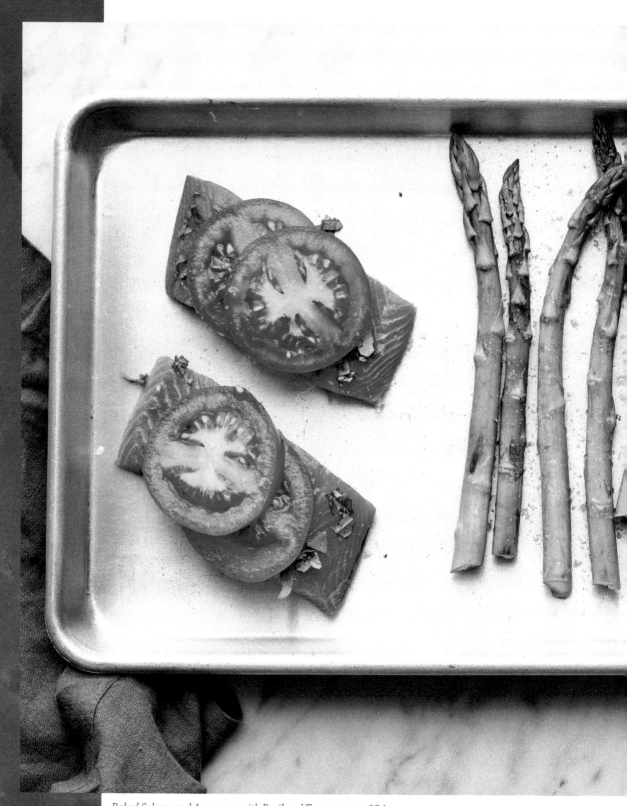

Baked Salmon and Asparagus with Basil and Tomato · page 124

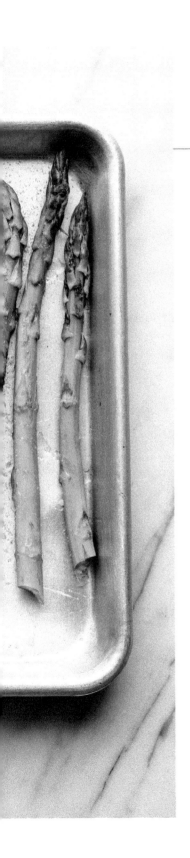

CHAPTER ONE

EATING MADE EASIER AFTER VSG

One of the most common questions I hear from patients after gastric sleeve surgery is "What do I eat?" This chapter will cover the details of vertical sleeve gastrectomy, how to prepare for surgery, and best practices for success after surgery, including what to eat for optimal healing and for living life with a sleeve.

The Benefits of Gastric Sleeve Surgery

Vertical sleeve gastrectomy (VSG) reduces the size of your stomach, restricting the amount of food you can eat and, therefore, decreasing your caloric intake, maximizing weight loss. Because of that weight loss, patients often find their health improved and that they can reduce or eliminate medications. I've seen conditions such as diabetes, hyperlipidemia, sleep apnea, infertility, and high blood pressure resolve naturally after surgery. Let's look at just a few of the major benefits of VSG.

» *Minimally invasive procedure.* Surgery usually takes just 40 to 70 minutes, and only a few small incisions are made. Compared to other bariatric surgery options, the recovery time is shorter, there is less post-op pain, and there is a much smaller risk of infection and scarring. The hospital stay is also typically short, with an average length of one to three days.

» *Automatic portion control.* VSG essentially downsizes the stomach, helping patients feel fuller with less food. The inability to eat the pre-surgery volume of food not only teaches patients how to eat reduced and healthy portion sizes but can also lead to natural weight loss. After time, this new portion sizing becomes a healthy habit.

» *Reduction in hunger.* Gastric sleeve surgery often reduces a person's desire for food because the part of the stomach that is removed is where the hunger hormone, ghrelin, is produced. This prevents overeating and helps patients choose food mindfully, not making decisions based on hunger alone.

» *Minimal dietary restrictions.* This procedure doesn't require a lot of modification of the patient's daily diet. Patients can choose from a variety of foods, which makes it easier to plan meals and cook. Only foods high in fat or added sugars are limited.

» *No malabsorption of food.* After surgery, your body will be able to take in many nutrients from the foods you eat and drink. Vitamin and mineral deficiencies are rare if patients supplement their diet with recommended vitamins and minerals.

VSG FAQS

In my work with patients and clients over the years, I've noticed the same questions come up repeatedly. Here are a few of the most common with my answers.

Q: *How fast will I lose weight after VSG?*
A: Most weight loss occurs in the first year. Keep in mind that for every patient, the weight loss amount, percentage, and timing are different. Some patients may need to lose more weight than others. The rate of weight loss depends on many factors including your activity level, gender, compliance, and preexisting conditions.

Q: *Will I ever be able to drink coffee again?*
A: According to the American Society of Metabolic and Bariatric Surgery (ASMBS), you should avoid caffeine for at least one month after surgery. Your stomach will be extra sensitive, and caffeine stimulates gastric acid secretion. Clarify with your surgeon or dietitian about when you will be allowed to reintroduce caffeinated drinks. When you start drinking coffee again, I suggest being highly aware of how much coffee creamer you add. Although some creamers are low-carb, they can be high in fat and calories. I also suggest not drinking very hot coffee, as it can damage the esophagus.

Q: *Does dumping syndrome occur with VSG?*
A: Dumping syndrome is when food is "dumped" directly from the stomach to the small intestine without being digested, causing bloating, cramps, diarrhea, nausea, and other ailments. It typically occurs after bariatric patients consume large amounts of high-sugar foods or a high-fat meal—but it's very rare after vertical sleeve gastrectomy. However, I've had patients assume that any gastrointestinal distress is a result of dumping syndrome. Many symptoms are similar. For example, diarrhea can be related to food poisoning, lactose intolerance, and medications. Vomiting can be a result of overeating or food poisoning. Gastrointestinal pain can be caused by foods high in sugar alcohol, the possible development of undiagnosed irritable bowel syndrome (IBS), or other undiagnosed underlying medical conditions.

Q: *Will my stomach stretch after surgery?*
A: After VSG, the stomach will stretch a little bit. The reason you eat less right after surgery is due to swelling in the area and slow motility (digestion). As

continued »

you recover, you will be able to drink and eat more because the food moves through and empties faster, but the stomach will never stretch back to its original size.

Q: *Can I exercise after VSG?*

A: Always consult your doctor before starting any type of physical activity. After surgery, you may feel tired, but moving is highly encouraged. Take it slowly, and try to establish healthy habits by moving whenever and however you can. Swimming and walking are great forms of exercise and easiest on the body in the beginning of recovery. Resistance training (or weight training) can help you build muscle and lose weight faster. Consider getting wrist or ankle weights, as these are a simple way to add resistance while doing your daily activities.

Food Without Fear After VSG

The first few weeks post-op will require you to focus on what you eat, how much you eat, and how often you eat as you heal and recover. But you will soon be able to transition to a lifelong way of eating and enjoying a variety of foods—just in smaller portions and with the appropriate balance of nutrients. The goal of this book is to help you make that transition as smoothly as possible. Let's look at some important ways you'll approach food and lifestyle after surgery.

UNDERSTANDING HUNGER AND CRAVINGS

Your body is smart. It knows how to take care of you and alert you to what it needs when it needs it. If you feel hungry, it's important to nourish your body with the food it needs to stay alive and function well. However, many of us have a hard time discerning between hunger and cravings. You will know you are truly hungry when you feel light-headed or irritable, have a headache, or have difficulty concentrating. Cravings aren't bad, but learning to manage them is key for lifelong weight maintenance. Here are a few best practices.

» *Understand your cravings.* Sometimes, it's okay to satisfy cravings. Constantly denying yourself a food you want or love isn't an enjoyable way to live. But always giving yourself over to cravings isn't the best option, either. When you feel a craving, ask yourself why you're craving that food. If you're craving it because you're stressed, anxious, sad, or lonely, ask yourself whether giving in to your craving will help solve this emotion or feeling. More often than not, it won't. Instead, find something to do other than eating to work through this emotion or experience: Call a friend, go for a walk, or read a book.

» *Eat well-balanced meals throughout the day.* After surgery, protein is the number-one nutrient your body needs. As you progress, you should eat a balance of proteins, carbohydrates, and fats. If you have complete meals with snacks in between, you will experience fewer cravings. Try to eat meals at regular, recurring times to prevent hunger, as doing so helps prevent overeating.

» *Drink water.* It's very important to stay hydrated during the weight-loss process. Sometimes people think they're hungry when, in reality, they are just thirsty.

MASTERING MEAL PLANNING AND MEAL PREPPING

Meal planning and meal prepping are helpful tools when it comes to eating healthy, balanced meals. By planning and being prepared, you will never need to reach for convenient, unhealthy, or fast foods. Here are a couple tips to make the most of meal planning and prepping.

» *Have a plan and stick to it.* First, look to see what ingredients you have on hand in the refrigerator, freezer, and pantry. Then create a list of what you would like to eat for breakfast, lunch, and dinner as well as for snacks. (Typically, you should eat every 3 to 4 hours.) Grocery shop for items you're missing and stick to your list—only buy what you need. And, of course, avoid shopping when you are hungry, as this can keep you from sticking to your plan.

» *Maximize your time in the kitchen.* As you cook, double or triple a recipe and store extras in the refrigerator or freezer so you have healthy meals to eat throughout the week without having to cook multiple times a day. I suggest purchasing a few glass storage containers of various sizes and plastic zip-top bags for storage (or silicone bags as they can be reused easily).

ADOPTING MINDFUL EATING

Practicing mindful eating—meaning eating with no distractions—is key to eating not only the right foods but also the right *amounts* of foods. Here are a few tips for eating more mindfully.

» *Take time to chew.* When you talk while eating, you may swallow extra air and may feel uncomfortable as a result. Instead, practice chewing your food slowly and thoroughly and try not to talk while eating.

» *Avoid distractions and focus on your plate.* Avoid eating while driving, watching TV, working on the computer, playing a game, looking at social media, or reading, as you will not be aware of what you're eating.

» *Don't eat while stressed.* It is very important not to eat when you experience stress or anxiety. Avoid eating during tense meetings at work or after a stressful event. Calm yourself using relaxation practices such as meditation, prayer, yoga, or breathing. There are a lot of free mobile apps that can help with relaxation; consider trying Calm or Headspace.

FINDING ENJOYMENT IN EATING

Many patients worry that they won't enjoy eating after VSG, but this is not the case. Although the first few weeks will be focused on consuming a mostly liquid and pureed foods diet, eventually you will be able to eat solid foods again, and you can enjoy most of your old favorite foods, just in moderation. Instead of thinking of this new way of eating as a chore, adopt a positive outlook about your new journey. Here are some ways to cultivate enjoyment around your new eating habits.

» *Try new things.* An easy way to get excited about what you eat is by trying new recipes. Bookmark recipes that are new to you and get you excited about cooking. Look at this as an opportunity to try new foods or ingredients you may never have tasted or cooked with before.

» *Embrace the social aspect of food.* Food isn't just fuel; it's also an opportunity to share an experience with others. Invite your friends or loved ones for a meal and cook some of your new favorite recipes or foods for them.

STRENGTHENING YOUR SELF-COMPASSION MUSCLE

Throughout this journey, it's important to be kind to yourself. Getting "off track" doesn't make you a failure; it makes you human. Here are two ways you can practice self-compassion.

» *Silence your inner critic.* Let go of any self-criticism and negative self-talk. Determine how you can be more kind, loving, and respectful toward yourself. Self-criticism will only provoke negative emotions and stress, which can cause overeating and prevent you from meeting your goals. Blaming and reprimanding yourself will only make you feel worse and affect your ability to think about the issue rationally.

» *Practice reciting positive and uplifting affirmations.* If you get off track, don't reprimand yourself. Just remind yourself that it's going to be a great day and you will improve next time.

SETTING YOURSELF UP FOR SUCCESS

Let's stop with the "diet" mentality. Sustainable, healthy weight loss is only possible when we develop lifelong healthy eating habits. Here are some other dieting mentalities I'd like you to consider removing from your life.

» *Ditch the scale.* Many patients want to buy a scale before or after surgery, but I discourage this. Getting on a scale every morning and seeing the numbers go up or down can cause a roller coaster of emotions. Your doctor will weigh you during your regular checkups. Oftentimes, patients become obsessed with the number on the scale. This is helpful information, but it does not tell the whole story. That number doesn't tell you the percentage of fat, muscle, excess skin, or water weight on your body. I suggest judging your success by how your clothes fit and other benefits of weight loss— things like no longer needing to take certain medications, resolving medical conditions, or requiring fewer doctor's visits.

» *Don't play the comparison game.* Remember: Some people may lose weight faster or slower than others. Don't compare your journey to the journeys of others.

Post-Op Nutrition at a Glance

Later in this book you will learn the four post-op dietary stages and find specific meal plans for each. In addition, I explain why certain dietary changes are important as you progress through the recovery stages and toward lifelong healthy eating. But first, let's cover the major food groups and the role each plays in your post-op diet.

While recovering from surgery during the first few months, it is very important to stay hydrated to prevent constipation, kidney stones, and dehydration. Dehydration is the most common reason for readmission to the hospital. Symptoms of dehydration include thirst, headache, constipation, or dizziness upon sitting or standing up. One way to tell if you're getting enough fluid it is to check the color of your urine, which should be a light color like lemonade, not dark like apple juice. You should urinate roughly five to 10 times per day.

I suggest carrying a reusable water bottle that you can refill throughout the day. Add flavor enhancers, such as basil, cucumber, or lemon, to keep from getting bored with plain water. Set reminders on your phone, place sticky notes on your computer or mirror, or ask a friend or family member to remind you to drink water.

Fluids should be consumed slowly, 30 minutes before or after meals, to prevent gastrointestinal distress. Avoid drinking from a water fountain or straw, as it is more difficult to control the volume of intake and doing so can introduce air into the stomach, causing gas, bloating, and abdominal discomfort.

What to drink: Water, decaf tea, noncarbonated sugar-free drinks, low-sodium tomato or vegetable juice, milk or unsweetened milk alternatives, low-sodium broth, sugar-free or low-sugar hot chocolate and ice pops.

Serving size: Drink a minimum of 64 ounces daily. More fluids may be needed when the temperature is high or with increased physical activity.

What to limit or avoid: For the first month after surgery, avoid drinks high in caffeine (coffee, energy drinks, soda, tea). It is generally okay to resume caffeine intake one month after surgery unless your doctor recommends otherwise. Also, as for long-term recommendations, avoid high-sugar drinks such as sodas and fruit juices (these are high in sugar and calories), carbonated drinks (these can cause increased gas, bloating, and discomfort), and spearmint or peppermint teas (which can cause heartburn due to acid reflux in some patients). Alcohol should be avoided entirely or limited.

PROTEIN

Protein is the most important macronutrient for patients who have undergone VSG. Your body needs it to maintain and build muscle, and it supports cellular and hormonal functions in the body. Your body cannot make protein on its own, which is why it's important to get enough from the foods you eat. When you don't take in enough protein, you may experience muscle loss, excessive hair loss, and hormonal abnormalities. Always start with the protein when eating a meal or snacks. To make sure you are consuming enough protein, I suggest tracking your daily intake. Stick with the recommended goal; excessive protein intake is not always beneficial.

After surgery you may need to supplement with protein shakes or powders for the first four to six months. Some patients continue to take smaller amounts of supplements indefinitely. You can purchase protein supplements in pharmacy stores, grocery stores, health nutrition food stores, and online. I suggest purchasing a few before your surgery so you are prepared. When choosing protein supplements, here's for what to look for:

1. *Choose whey protein isolate.* This is one of the highest-quality protein powders. If you are lactose intolerant, avoid whey concentrate unless taken with lactase pills. Lactose can cause digestive distress such as bloating, gas, or diarrhea in some patients after surgery, so avoid whey if you experience these symptoms.

2. *Consider nondairy protein supplements.* If you are allergic or intolerant to whey, consider egg protein powder or plant-based protein powders like the ones made from soy or peas.

3. *Avoid hydrolyzed protein supplements.* Hydrolyzed protein supplements, like gelatin or collagen proteins, may be of lesser quality or not a complete protein.

4. *Pick supplements low in sugar and fat.* Read the label carefully; sometimes protein supplements can have a lot of added sugar. Generally, opt for protein powders with 10 to 20 grams of protein per serving, 5 to 10 grams or less of added sugars, and 5 grams or less of fat. Milk-based protein supplements typically have natural milk sugar from lactose.

What to eat: Preferable sources of protein are lean meats such as chicken, fish, or turkey; eggs; nonfat dairy such as milk, yogurt, kefir, cottage cheese, and low-fat cheese; and vegetarian sources of protein such as beans, lentils, tofu, nuts, seeds, and soy. Lean cuts of red meat should be consumed less often.

Serving size: The generally recommended amounts of daily protein consumption are a minimum of 60 to 80 grams for women and 70 to 90 grams for men. Check with your medical team about your specific daily protein goal and calculate your protein intake to make sure you get enough but not too much.

What to limit or avoid: Limit high-fat dairy and high-fat red meat (beef, lamb, pork). Avoid grilled or smoked meats and processed meats (bacon, hot dogs, lunch meats) because these foods have added nitrates, which can damage the lining of the gut and can increase the risk for chronic diseases such as colorectal cancer.

CARBOHYDRATES

Carbohydrates are a very important macronutrient, the main source of energy for the body, and the body's primary source of fuel for the brain. That is why, when hungry, you feel light-headed or have a headache. A lot of patients avoid all carbs, but that is not a healthy solution. Your liver stores carbohydrates in the form of glycogen (sugar), which helps control blood sugar while sleeping. We need to eat carbohydrates every day to restore that energy. Long-term high-protein, low-carbohydrate diets can also cause muscle loss because the body uses protein as energy when not enough carbohydrates are available.

There are two types of carbs: simple and complex. Simple carbohydrates include refined white flour, candy, juice, and other processed foods that are quickly burned by the body for fuel. Complex carbohydrates, as from fruits, vegetables, and whole grains, are full of other nutrients, minerals, and fiber and break down in the body more slowly, providing a steady source of energy without the blood sugar spike and crash often associated with eating simple carbs. Hypoglycemia (low blood sugar) can occur a few months after surgery, generally a result of not consuming enough carbohydrates throughout the day. Combine protein and carbohydrates at each meal, especially if you exercise regularly, as the body needs to refuel and repair itself after physical activity.

What to eat: High-fiber carbohydrates such as whole grains (buckwheat, farro, oats, quinoa, wild rice); vegetables such as corn, peas, potatoes, and yams; fruits; and nonfat dairy (kefir, milk, yogurt), which contains natural sugars.

Serving size: Bariatric patients do not need to count carbs unless they are diabetic and on insulin. Pairing proper protein consumption with a variety of dairy, fruit, grain, and vegetable options will ensure that you get enough carbohydrates. Try to consume less than 5 to 7 grams of added sugar per meal.

What to limit or avoid: Syrups, white or brown sugar, fruit juice, candy, and soda should be avoided or limited due to their very high added-sugar content. Be careful when eating doughy breads, pastas, and rice, as they are not easily tolerated for several months after surgery.

FAT

Fat is another important macronutrient. When you don't consume enough fat, you may feel tired, hungry, and weak or notice dry skin and low energy. Your body cannot make essential fatty acids like omega-3 and omega-6, and for a few weeks after surgery, it may be hard to get enough fat in your diet. For this reason, I include avocado, nut butters, and olive oil in the recipes in this book, even in the first stages of the diet to prevent fatty acid deficiency.

It is very important to distinguish between unhealthy saturated fats and healthy unsaturated fats. Saturated fats are mostly found in animal products such as butter and margarine, chicken, dairy, and meat. Plant-based sources of saturated fats include coconut oil and palm oil. These should be avoided or consumed in small amounts only. In my recipes, you will find suggestions for choosing low-fat or nonfat dairy and lean cuts of meat.

Unsaturated fats, also called monounsaturated or polyunsaturated fats, are mostly found in avocado, fish, nuts, olives, and seeds. Some of the best oils for cooking are olive oil, canola oil, and avocado oil. Following is a quick cheat sheet for choosing healthy fats when cooking after VSG.

INSTEAD OF	USE
Butter or margarine	Avocado oil, canola oil, grape-seed oil, olive oil, and sesame oil
Sour cream	Greek yogurt (plain, nonfat, or 2%)
Mayonnaise	Light mayonnaise or mustard

What to eat: Avocado, fish, nuts and seeds and their butters, olive oil, and vegetable oil.

Serving size: 30 percent of total calories should come from fat and 7 percent of that should be saturated fat.

What to limit or avoid: Avoid high-fat dairy, high-fat red meats, fried foods, greasy or oily foods, fast foods, and palm and coconut oil.

SUPPLEMENTATION

Supplementation to avoid nutrient deficiencies is critical after VSG, and most patients will need to supplement for the rest of their lives. After gastric sleeve surgery, you may not be able to eat a variety of foods due to personal preference and tolerance, volume restriction, or other reasons. There is also the possibility of impaired absorption of some nutrients. For this reason, supplementation is crucial. Failing to take additional amounts of these nutrients could lead to medical problems.

In my years of practice, I have met many gastric sleeve patients who don't supplement correctly or don't take any supplements at all. Some have had serious vitamin and mineral deficiencies and have suffered memory loss, severe hair loss, dry skin, damaged nails, and neurological deficiencies, to name a few problems. I've heard many excuses for why patients do not take supplements: forgetfulness, financial restraints, lack of direction from their medical provider, or the belief that supplements aren't necessary.

I highly suggest consuming quality supplements made especially for patients who have had gastric sleeve surgery. Over-the-counter products made for the general population may not contain all the needed nutrients. The recommendations established by the ASMBS are two complete multivitamins with minerals and iron. (Some patients may need additional iron depending on blood work.) It is important also to supplement with vitamins B_{12} and D and calcium. (Some patients may also need an additional B complex.) I list reputable supplement companies in the Resources section (see page 175).

Tips for supplementation after surgery:

» For the first few months, choose liquid, chewable, crushable, or sprayable forms of supplements. As recovery progresses, you can transition to pills or capsules.

» Consult your surgical team on when you can begin supplementation. For the first few days it may be difficult to take supplements due to volume restriction, taste, or nausea. Some surgeons recommended avoiding supplements for several days after surgery.

» Take multivitamin supplements with food for better absorption and tolerance.

» You may get B_{12} in sublingual form (a pill that is placed under the tongue), as injections, or as a nasal spray.

» Calcium citrate is preferred. Pills can be crushed and then dissolved in a small amount of water or a sugar-free drink. Do not take more than 500 mg of calcium at a time. And do not take calcium with your iron supplement, as calcium can interfere with iron absorption.

» Iron may be needed for the first few months after surgery, and blood work needs to be monitored to determine if supplementation is necessary. Avoid taking iron with acid-reducing medication, calcium supplements, milk, calcium-fortified drinks, coffee, or tea, as they decrease the absorption of iron. Wait two to three hours to consume iron after consuming calcium.

» Avoid gummy or children's supplements, as they may not be complete.

ALCOHOL AND SWEETENERS

» *Alcohol.* Alcohol is typically not recommended after VSG. First, alcohol has no nutritional value—that's why you will not see nutrition facts labels on alcoholic products. Alcohol is also high in calories: Alcoholic cocktails can range between 200 and 600 calories. Alcohol can also cause stomach and intestinal discomfort resulting in pain, cramping, and diarrhea.

» *Sugar alcohols.* I highly recommend carefully reading labels and paying attention to sugar alcohols. These include erythritol, lactitol, maltitol, mannitol, sorbitol, and xylitol. Sugar alcohol lurks in foods like protein drinks and bars, bariatric supplements, and sugar-free candies. I suggest no more than 5 to 10 grams of sugar alcohol per serving. High amounts of sugar alcohol can lead to abdominal pain, bloating, cramping, diarrhea, and a lot of gas.

» *High-intensity sweeteners.* Sugar substitutes can be used after surgery. Some patients may want to use sugar-free syrups or sugar-free sweeteners to sweeten coffee, tea, and other foods. In the United States, there are eight sugar substitutes permitted for use in food: acesulfame-K, advantame, aspartame, monk fruit, neotame, saccharine, stevia, and sucralose. Although I don't advise in favor of or against any, if you prefer not to use sugar substitutes, I suggest using natural sources of sugar such as honey in very small amounts, about 1 to 2 teaspoons per serving. If you use white or brown sugar, cane sugar, or agave syrup, consume no more than 5 grams per serving.

EATING OUT MADE EASIER

For the first few weeks, and possibly months, following surgery, most of your meals will be made at home. However, dining out with friends and family is an important part of enjoying an active social life. These tips can help you make the healthiest food choices so you can leave the restaurant feeling satisfied.

Tip 1: *Plan ahead*. Before you go, do some research. Most restaurants have an online menu you can preview before you arrive. You will have less anxiety about what to eat when you know your options ahead of time.

Tip 2: *Ask for condiments on the side*. Ask for condiments such as butter, margarine, creamy sauces, dressings, or sour cream on the side. Avoid or eat only small amounts of ranch dressing, mayonnaise, tartar sauce, or any other creamy condiments. Whenever possible, choose condiments low in calories and fats, such as balsamic vinegar, mustard, relish, or salsa.

Tip 3: *Order a kid's meal or ask for a to-go box*. If the restaurant will allow it, order from the kid's menu. Typically, a kid's meal offers smaller portions of food and comes with the option of healthy sides such as fruits or vegetables. If this is not possible, ask your server for a to-go box when your meal arrives. Pack up half of your meal to go so you're not temped to eat it all at one sitting.

Tip 4: *Pay attention to certain words on the menu*. Look for words like *broiled, garden fresh, roasted*, and *steamed*, which often indicate healthier cooking methods. Be cautious with dishes that include words like *breaded, butter sauce, cheesy, cream sauce, fried, sautéed*, and *tempura*. Typically, these foods are high in fat and calories.

Tip 5: *Go for the macronutrients*. Choose a dish with a lean protein, such as chicken, fish, shrimp, or turkey, or plant-based protein like beans or tofu. Then choose a side of healthy carbohydrates, such as buckwheat, corn, quinoa, or yams, and a side of vegetables (steamed or grilled) or a salad with dressing on the side.

About the Book's Recipes

When I set out to write this book, I wanted to make sure the recipes were easy to make and nutritionally balanced for your post-surgery needs. But more than that, I want you to enjoy the food you eat, and I promise the delicious recipes in this book will help you do just that. All the recipes call for just a few familiar ingredients, don't require long prep or clean-up times, and will help you on the road to weight loss and healthy weight maintenance—without sacrificing taste or flavor. These recipes call for real food ingredients to assist you toward sustainable weight loss as well as help prevent or even reverse chronic conditions on your way to enjoying a healthy, delicious life.

Some recipes yield one serving, but you can always double a recipe and store the leftovers. I have included storage tips for those that store well so you can enjoy delicious, healthy options whenever you're hungry or even when you don't feel like cooking. I have also put together meal plans and shopping lists in chapter 2, which will help guide you through the stages of recovery into a life of healthy eating habits.

UNDERSTANDING LABELS

These recipes were created with ease in mind. Thus, you will see a variety of labels on a majority of the recipes indicating how they fulfill that promise. They are:

» *5 Ingredients or Fewer:* The recipe requires five or fewer ingredients—excluding salt, pepper, water, and oil.

» *30 Minutes or Less:* The recipe takes less than 30 minutes from start to finish, including prepping ingredients.

» *No Cook:* The recipe requires zero heat or active cooking time, only assembly.

» *One Pot:* The recipe uses one vessel to prepare and cook the meal.

KEY FEATURES FOR SUCCESS

Along with the easy labels featured, each recipe includes a few key tools to help you navigate post-op sleeve eating.

» *Post-op portion size.* Although the stomach size of each patient will differ, each recipe indicates the suggested serving size based on the recovery stage for which the recipe is intended. Keep in mind that it may take you a while to drink or eat a meal: It may take up to an hour to sip a shake. As time goes by, you will be able to tolerate more volume in less time. But you don't have to consume the whole drink or meal. Stop when you feel full and save the rest for another time.

» *Helpful recipe headnotes and tips.* In the recipe headnotes, you will learn the reason for the recipe being included in the book or the specific stage, ingredient swaps for variations on the recipe, and other helpful information. At the end of many recipes, you will find a tip to help you better prepare, cook, eat, or store meals for future use or how to mix things up. I also include post-op tips wherever appropriate. I recommend reading the recipes as you review the meal plans and before grocery shopping, as you may find alternatives or ingredient swaps that appeal to your palate preferences or dietary needs.

» *Nutritional information.* Each recipe includes key nutritional information, including total calories and grams of protein, carbs, fat, sugar, and added sugar.

NECESSARY EQUIPMENT AND TOOLS

To successfully prepare your post-op meals, you will need some equipment and tools, many of which you probably have but some that you may need to invest in. These tools will make the transition to a VSG diet much easier and make your new lifestyle sustainable for the long term. Keep in mind that you won't be spending as much money on groceries because you will be eating less and you're investing in kitchen tools that can last a long time and make cooking easy and fun.

» Aluminum foil, nonstick
» Baking dishes (glass or ceramic)
» Baking sheets and sheet pans
» Blender
» Cutting board
» Food scale
» Glass storage containers (varying sizes)
» Measuring cups and spoons (for dry and liquid ingredients)
» Mini food processor
» Mixing bowls (small, medium, and large)
» Muffin tins
» Parchment paper
» Plastic or silicone zip-top storage bags (varying sizes)
» Plastic wrap
» Pots and pans with lids (varying sizes)
» Ramekins (6 ounces)
» Sharp knife
» Spatula, whisk, tongs, mixing spoons

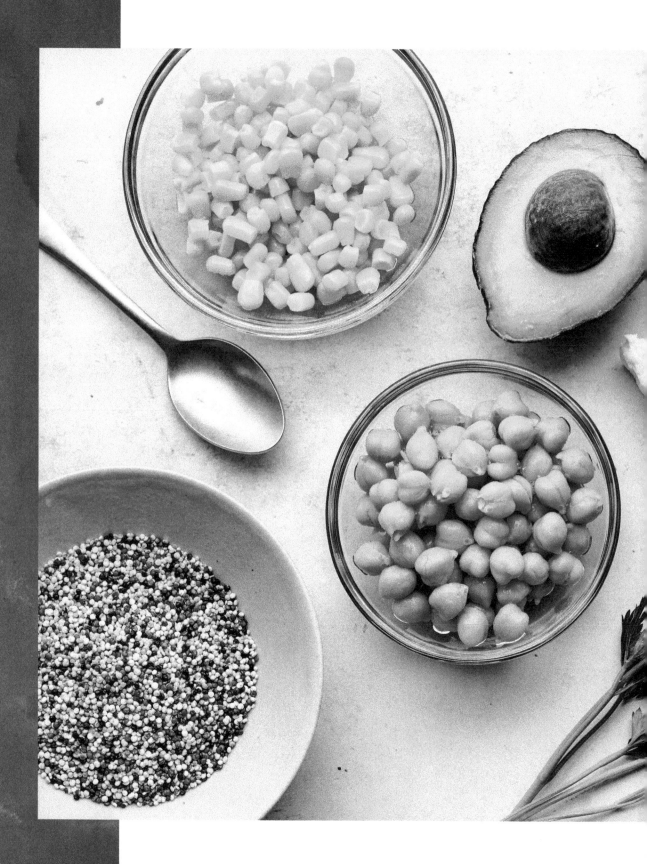

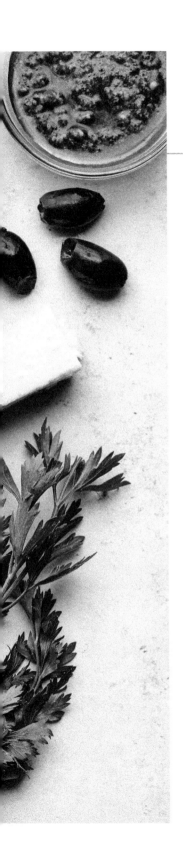

CHAPTER TWO

YOUR POST-OP MEAL PLAN

In this chapter, you will find a stage-by-stage meal plan for eating in the weeks following gastric sleeve surgery. By following a meal plan, you can save money, save time in the kitchen, and waste less food. There are also grocery lists for each stage to make meal planning as easy as possible.

Four Stages to Healing

Over the next few weeks, use this book's meal plans to guide you on the road to recovery and lifelong eating after VSG. I suggest keeping a food journal to track your protein intake and hydration and any symptoms you experience as you reintroduce foods.

For the first week or two, you will be on a full liquid diet. You will then progress to pureed foods, then to a soft foods diet, and eventually to solid foods. However, you can always go back and eat liquid, pureed, or soft foods at any time once you've completed those stages if it fits your lifestyle and preferences.

Before you begin each stage, read the recipes to see what you will be eating. Each recipe contains suggestions for swapping or varying ingredients to give you options for your personal preference or needs, variety, and more meal ideas. Just be sure to update your grocery list accordingly. I include staple ingredients, like olive oil and spices, across all grocery lists, but you do not need to rebuy these each week if you have an ample supply.

Please note: Each person is different, and every recovery period is different. The length recommendations for the stages are the general standard for most patients. Always consult your surgeon and dietitian about your progress before moving to the next stage to determine what is best for you.

STAGE 1: LIQUID DIET (WEEKS 1 TO 2)

A liquid diet means you are allowed liquefied foods with the consistency of milk, yogurt, or pudding. Use a blender to achieve a smooth consistency and a strainer to make sure there are no chunks remaining.

During the liquid diet stage, it is crucial that you stay hydrated and get the recommended amount of protein. The meal plan that follows is designed to help you do this by consuming shakes, smoothies, and soups. You can also purchase unflavored protein powder to add to your shakes and smoothies in this stage and beyond. Although soups are not high in protein, they are a great savory liquid meal option. It's also critical to consume the proper amount of fatty acids, which is why I include recipes made with healthy fats.

Some surgeons and dietitians may instruct you not to take vitamins for the first few days post-op due to possible poor tolerance. This is why I include commercial protein drinks which are meal replacements fortified with vitamins and nutrients, across the meal plans.

Typically, patients follow this diet for one or two weeks after surgery. I provide two weeks here, if needed. When you think you are ready to progress to the next stage, consult your surgeon and bariatric dietitian.

Week 1 Meal Plan: Liquid Diet

	BREAKFAST	SNACK	LUNCH	SNACK	DINNER	SNACK
MONDAY	Commercial protein shake	Cinnamon-Vanilla Kefir Shake (page 51)	Commercial protein shake	5 ounces nonfat plain Greek yogurt or Icelandic-style skyr	Tomato-Avocado Juice (page 55)	8 ounces nonfat kefir
TUESDAY	Commercial protein shake	Soy Chocolate Milk Shake (page 52)	Commercial protein shake	5 ounces nonfat plain Greek yogurt or Icelandic-style skyr	Easy Butternut Squash Soup (page 56)	8 ounces nonfat kefir
WEDNESDAY	Commercial protein shake	Banana Yogurt Shake (page 54)	Commercial protein shake	5 ounces nonfat plain Greek yogurt or Icelandic-style skyr	*Leftover* Easy Butternut Squash Soup	Nut Butter Ice Pops (page 49)
THURSDAY	Commercial protein shake	Cinnamon-Vanilla Kefir Shake (page 51)	Commercial protein shake	5 ounces nonfat plain Greek yogurt or Icelandic-style skyr	*Leftover* Easy Butternut Squash Soup	*Leftover* Nut Butter Ice Pops
FRIDAY	Commercial protein shake	Soy Chocolate Milk Shake (page 52)	Commercial protein shake	5 ounces nonfat plain Greek yogurt or Icelandic-style skyr	*Leftover* Easy Butternut Squash Soup	8 ounces nonfat kefir
SATURDAY	Commercial protein shake	Banana Yogurt Shake (page 54)	Commercial protein shake	5 ounces nonfat plain Greek yogurt or Icelandic-style skyr	Tomato-Avocado Juice (page 55)	*Leftover* Nut Butter Ice Pops
SUNDAY	Commercial protein shake	Banana Yogurt Shake (page 54)	Commercial protein shake	5 ounces nonfat plain Greek yogurt or Icelandic-style skyr	Tomato-Avocado Juice (page 55)	*Leftover* Nut Butter Ice Pops

Week 1 Grocery List: Liquid Diet

PRODUCE

» Avocado *(1)*
» Bananas *(4)*
» Butternut squash *(10 ounces fresh, or 1 [10-ounce] bag, frozen)*
» Chives *(1 bunch; optional)*
» Parsley *(1 bunch)*

DAIRY AND NONDAIRY ALTERNATIVES

» Almond milk, unsweetened *(12 ounces); I prefer Orgain Brand Organic Protein*
» Greek yogurt or Icelandic-style skyr, nonfat plain *(7 [5-ounce] containers)*, plus Greek yogurt, nonfat plain *(3 cups)*
» Ice cream, sugar-free vanilla *(8 ounces)*
» Kefir, nonfat plain *(40 ounces)*
» Soy milk, unsweetened *(16 ounces)*

PANTRY

DRIED HERBS AND SPICES

» Black pepper, freshly ground
» Cinnamon, ground
» Salt
» Vanilla extract

BOTTLED, CANNED, JARRED, AND PACKAGED

» Almond butter, creamy, no added sugar
» Broth, low-sodium chicken *(12 ounces)*
» Honey; *Manuka is one of the best-quality types*
» Oil, olive
» Syrup, sugar-free chocolate; *I prefer Torani brand of syrup*
» Syrup, sugar-free, or sugar-free sweetener

OTHER

» Protein shakes, commercial, at least 15 to 30 grams protein *(14)*
» Tomato juice, low-sodium *(24 ounces)*

Week 2 Meal Plan: Liquid Diet

	BREAKFAST	SNACK	LUNCH	SNACK	DINNER	SNACK
MONDAY	Commercial protein shake	Creamy Chocolate Shake (page 50)	Commercial protein shake	5 ounces nonfat plain Greek yogurt or Icelandic-style skyr	Tomato-Avocado Juice (page 55)	8 ounces nonfat kefir
TUESDAY	Commercial protein shake	Triple Almond Shake (page 53)	Commercial protein shake	5 ounces nonfat plain Greek yogurt or Icelandic-style skyr	Tomato-Avocado Juice (page 55)	8 ounces nonfat kefir
WEDNESDAY	Commercial protein shake	Banana Yogurt Shake (page 54)	Commercial protein shake	5 ounces nonfat plain Greek yogurt or Icelandic-style skyr	Tomato-Avocado Juice (page 55)	8 ounces nonfat milk
THURSDAY	Commercial protein shake	Creamy Chocolate Shake (page 50)	Commercial protein shake	5 ounces nonfat plain Greek yogurt or Icelandic-style skyr	Tomato-Avocado Juice (page 55)	8 ounces nonfat kefir
FRIDAY	Commercial protein shake	Triple Almond Shake (page 53)	Commercial protein shake	5 ounces nonfat plain Greek yogurt or Icelandic-style skyr	Tomato-Avocado Juice (page 55)	8 ounces nonfat milk
SATURDAY	Commercial protein shake	Creamy Chocolate Shake (page 50)	Commercial protein shake	5 ounces nonfat plain Greek yogurt or Icelandic-style skyr	Tomato-Avocado Juice (page 55)	High-Protein Hot Chocolate Milk (page 48)
SUNDAY	Commercial protein shake	Banana Yogurt Shake (page 54)	Commercial protein shake	5 ounces nonfat plain Greek yogurt or Icelandic-style skyr	Tomato-Avocado Juice (page 55)	High-Protein Hot Chocolate Milk (page 48)

Week 2 Grocery List: Liquid Diet

PRODUCE
» Avocados *(2)*
» Banana *(1)*
» Chives *(1 bunch; optional)*
» Parsley *(1 bunch)*

DAIRY AND NONDAIRY ALTERNATIVES
» Almond milk, unsweetened *(24 ounces)*
» Creamer, vanilla *(2 tablespoons; optional)*
» Greek yogurt, nonfat plain, or Icelandic-style skyr *(7 [5-ounce]* containers)*, plus Greek yogurt, nonfat plain *(1 cup)*
» Kefir, nonfat plain *(24 ounces)*
» Milk, nonfat *(half gallon)*; I prefer Fairlife brand*

PANTRY
DRIED HERBS AND SPICES
» Black pepper, freshly ground
» Coconut extract
» Salt
» Vanilla extract

BOTTLED, CANNED, JARRED, AND PACKAGED
» Almond butter, creamy, no added sugar
» Almond powder *(1 [16-ounce] bag)*; I prefer Noosh brand*
» Cacao powder, unsweetened
» Dry milk powder, nonfat; *I prefer Carnation brand*
» Oil, olive
» Syrup, sugar-free vanilla, or sugar-free sweetener

OTHER
» Protein shakes, commercial, with at least 15 to 30 grams of protein *(14)*
» Tomato juice, low-sodium *(56 ounces)*

STAGE 2: PUREED FOODS *(WEEKS 3 TO 4)*

During the pureed phase, you will focus on meeting your protein needs, getting enough hydration, and reintroducing texture to your diet as you progress toward eating solid foods. As with the liquid diet, it may be difficult to get enough protein during this stage, so it is important to track your protein intake and follow the meal plan as directed. Although you may tolerate other foods, this diet is designed to give your body time to heal and adjust after surgery and lessen the chance of developing complications. You should continue supplementing with commercial protein drinks to make sure you get enough protein.

A blender or food processor will be an essential part of your meal prep, as will the use of measuring cups and spoons and a kitchen scale to ensure proper portions, which will help you adjust to monitoring portion sizes.

Typically, patients follow this diet for one or two weeks. When you think you are ready to progress to the next stage, consult your surgeon or bariatric dietitian.

Week 1 Meal Plan: Pureed Foods

	BREAKFAST	SNACK	LUNCH	SNACK	DINNER	SNACK
MONDAY	Baked Cinnamon-Apple Ricotta (page 66, *double the recipe*)	Commercial protein shake	¼ cup nonfat cottage cheese + 4 ounces no-sugar-added applesauce	Commercial protein shake	Easy Green Pea and Ham Soup (page 68, *freeze 1 portion for Week 2: Pureed Foods*)	5 ounces nonfat plain Greek yogurt
TUESDAY	*Leftover* Baked Cinnamon-Apple Ricotta	Commercial protein shake	5 ounces nonfat plain Greek yogurt	Commercial protein shake	*Leftover* Easy Green Pea and Ham Soup	8 ounces nonfat kefir
WEDNESDAY	Nutty Creamy Wheat Bowl (page 65)	Commercial protein shake	¼ cup nonfat cottage cheese + 4 ounces no-sugar-added applesauce	Commercial protein shake	*Leftover* Easy Green Pea and Ham Soup	5 ounces nonfat plain Greek yogurt
THURSDAY	Piña Colada Smoothie (page 62)	Commercial protein shake	5 ounces nonfat plain Greek yogurt	Commercial protein shake	*Leftover* Easy Green Pea and Ham Soup	8 ounces nonfat kefir
FRIDAY	Piña Colada Smoothie (page 62)	Commercial protein shake	Savory Chicken Salad (page 69)	Commercial protein shake	Decadent Tomato-Basil Soup (page 67)	Peachy Greek Yogurt Panna Cotta (page 64)
SATURDAY	Nutty Creamy Wheat Bowl (page 65)	Commercial protein shake	*Leftover* Savory Chicken Salad	Commercial protein shake	*Leftover* Decadent Tomato-Basil Soup	*Leftover* Peachy Greek Yogurt Panna Cotta
SUNDAY	Piña Colada Smoothie (page 62)	Commercial protein shake	*Leftover* Savory Chicken Salad	Commercial protein shake	*Leftover* Decadent Tomato-Basil Soup	*Leftover* Peachy Greek Yogurt Panna Cotta

Week 1 Grocery List: Pureed Foods

PRODUCE
» Banana *(1)*
» Onion, purple *(1)*
» Parsley *(1 small bunch)*
» Scallion *(1)* or chives
  (1 small bunch)

FROZEN FOODS
» Peas *(1 [10-ounce] package)*

DAIRY AND NONDAIRY ALTERNATIVES
» Coconut milk, unsweetened
  (12 ounces); *do not buy canned*
» Cheese, cottage, nonfat, no added
  salt *(½ cup)*; *I prefer Muuna, Good
  Culture, and Lifeway brands, or
  farmer's-style cottage cheese*
» Greek yogurt, nonfat plain *(7 cups)*
» Kefir, nonfat plain *(16 ounces)*
» Milk, nonfat *(12 ounces)*
» Ricotta, part skim *(1 cup)*

MEAT
» Ham or Canadian bacon, uncured, no nitrates added *(4 ounces)*

PANTRY
DRIED HERBS AND SPICES
» Basil
» Black pepper,
  freshly ground
» Cinnamon, ground
» Coconut extract
» Garlic powder
» Nutmeg, ground
» Onion powder
» Salt
» Vanilla extract

BOTTLED, CANNED, JARRED, AND PACKAGED
» Almond butter, creamy,
  no added sugar
» Applesauce, no sugar
  added *(1½ cups)*
» Chicken, low sodium
  (1 [12-ounce] can)
» Broth, low-sodium
  chicken *(20 ounces)*
» Cream of Wheat
  (1 [28-ounce] package)
» Gelatin, unflavored powder
» Honey
» Oil, olive
» Pineapple, chunks, no sugar
  added *(2 [15-ounce] cans)*
» Peaches, sliced, no sugar added
  (1 [14.5-ounce] can)
» Tomatoes, low-sodium whole or
  diced *(1 [15-ounce] can)*
» Vinegar, aged balsamic

OTHER
» Protein shakes, commercial, at least 15 to 30 grams protein *(14)*

Week 2 Meal Plan: Pureed Foods

	BREAKFAST	SNACK	LUNCH	SNACK	DINNER	SNACK
MONDAY	Green Mango Smoothie (page 63)	Commercial protein shake	*Leftover (from Week 1: Pureed Foods)* Savory Chicken Salad	Commercial protein shake	*Leftover (from Week 1: Pureed Foods)* Decadent Tomato-Basil Soup	*Leftover* Peachy Greek Yogurt Panna Cotta
TUESDAY	Herb and Melon Kefir Smoothie (page 60)	Commercial protein shake	¼ cup nonfat cottage cheese + 4 ounces no-sugar-added applesauce	Commercial protein shake	*Leftover* Easy Green Pea and Ham Soup (thawed)	5 ounces nonfat plain Greek yogurt
WEDNESDAY	Kefir and Yogurt Banana Flaxseed Shake (page 61)	Commercial protein shake	¼ cup nonfat cottage cheese + 4 ounces no-sugar-added applesauce	Commercial protein shake	¼ cup tuna + 1 teaspoon light mayonnaise	8 ounces nonfat kefir
THURSDAY	Nutty Creamy Wheat Bowl (page 65)	Commercial protein shake	Baked Cinnamon-Apple Ricotta (page 66, *triple the recipe*)	Commercial protein shake	¼ tuna + 1 teaspoon light mayonnaise	5 ounces nonfat plain Greek yogurt
FRIDAY	Green Mango Smoothie (page 63)	Commercial protein shake	*Leftover* Baked Cinnamon-Apple Ricotta	Commercial protein shake	Savory Chicken Salad (page 69)	8 ounces nonfat kefir
SATURDAY	Herb and Melon Kefir Smoothie (page 60)	Commercial protein shake	¼ cup nonfat cottage cheese + 4 ounces no-sugar-added applesauce	Commercial protein shake	*Leftover* Savory Chicken Salad	5 ounces nonfat plain Greek yogurt
SUNDAY	Kefir and Yogurt Banana Flaxseed Shake (page 61)	Commercial protein shake	*Leftover* Baked Cinnamon-Apple Ricotta	Commercial protein shake	*Leftover* Savory Chicken Salad	8 ounces nonfat kefir

Week 2 Grocery List: Pureed Foods

PRODUCE
» Avocado *(1)*
» Bananas *(2)*
» Basil *(1 small container)*
» Dill *(1 small container; optional)*
» Honeydew *(1)*
» Mint *(1 small container)*
» Scallion *(1)* or chives *(1 small bunch)*
» Spinach *(1 ounce)*

DAIRY AND NONDAIRY ALTERNATIVES
» Cheese, cottage, nonfat, no added salt *(¾ cup)*
» Greek yogurt, nonfat plain *(6 cups)*
» Kefir, nonfat plain *(5 cups)*
» Milk, nonfat *(1½ cups)*
» Ricotta, part skim *(1½ cups)*

PANTRY
DRIED HERBS AND SPICES
» Black pepper, freshly ground
» Cinnamon, ground
» Flaxseed, ground
» Garlic powder
» Nutmeg, ground
» Onion powder
» Salt
» Vanilla extract

BOTTLED, CANNED, JARRED, AND PACKAGED
» Almond butter, creamy, no added sugar
» Applesauce, no sugar added *(2½ cups)*
» Chicken, low sodium *(1 [12-ounce] can)*
» Honey
» Mango, chunks, no sugar added *(1 [15-ounce] can)*
» Mayonnaise, light
» Sunflower seed butter, creamy, no salt added
» Syrup, sugar-free vanilla
» Tuna *(2 [5-ounce] cans)*

OTHER
» Protein powder, unflavored; *I prefer Unjury or Beneprotein by Nestle brands*
» Protein shakes, commercial, at least 15 to 30 grams protein *(14)*

I like to call this stage "easy-to-digest foods." Here, you will slowly start to expand your food list by incorporating meals from the pureed foods diet, like Savory Chicken Salad (page 69), as well as commercial protein shakes, into a week of soft-food recipes. Be certain to maintain adequate hydration. Avoid a high intake of fibrous foods to allow for continued healing, and introduce soft solid foods slowly. Remember: Do not eat and drink at the same time to avoid overfilling the stomach and resulting discomfort, and chew food thoroughly.

Typically, patients follow this diet for two to four weeks. I include a two-week meal plan here, but you can repeat these meals as necessary. When you think you are ready to progress to the next stage, consult your surgeon or bariatric dietitian.

Week 1 Meal Plan: Soft Diet

	BREAKFAST	SNACK	LUNCH	SNACK	DINNER	SNACK
MONDAY	Rise-and-Shine Breakfast Soufflé (page 72, *double the recipe*)	Commercial protein shake	*Leftover (from Week 2: Pureed Foods)* Savory Chicken Salad	Commercial protein shake	Ricotta with Tomato Sauce and Parmesan (page 78, *triple the recipe*)	8 ounces nonfat kefir
TUESDAY	*Leftover* Rise-and-Shine Breakfast Soufflé	Commercial protein shake	Savory Chicken Salad (page 69)	Commercial protein shake	*Leftover* Ricotta with Tomato Sauce and Parmesan	5 ounces nonfat plain Greek yogurt
WEDNESDAY	Beans and Cheese with Avocado (page 79, *double the recipe*)	Commercial protein shake	*Leftover* Ricotta with Tomato Sauce and Parmesan	Commercial protein shake	*Leftover* Savory Chicken Salad	8 ounces nonfat milk
THURSDAY	*Leftover* Beans and Cheese with Avocado	Commercial protein shake	Scallion and Mustard Egg Salad (page 76)	Commercial protein shake	*Leftover* Savory Chicken Salad	8 ounces nonfat kefir
FRIDAY	Baked Ricotta and Banana with Nut Butter (page 73, *triple the recipe*)	Commercial protein shake	Tuna-Avocado Salad (page 80)	Commercial protein shake	*Leftover* Savory Chicken Salad	5 ounces nonfat plain Greek yogurt
SATURDAY	*Leftover* Baked Ricotta and Banana with Nut Butter	Commercial protein shake	Soft Basil Pesto Chicken (page 84)	Commercial protein shake	*Leftover* Scallion and Mustard Egg Salad	8 ounces nonfat milk
SUNDAY	*Leftover* Baked Ricotta and Banana with Nut Butter	Commercial protein shake	*Leftover* Tuna-Avocado Salad	Commercial protein shake	*Leftover* Soft Basil Pesto Chicken	8 ounces nonfat kefir

Week 1 Grocery List: Soft Diet

PRODUCE

» Avocados *(2)*
» Bananas *(2)*
» Basil *(1 small container; optional)*
» Dill *(1 small container; optional)*
» Lemon *(1)*
» Scallions *(2)* or chives *(1 small bunch)*
» Tomato *(1)*

DAIRY, NONDAIRY ALTERNATIVES, AND EGGS

» Cheese, Cheddar, low fat, shredded *(1 [8-ounce] bag)*
» Cheese, Parmesan, shredded or shaved *(3 tablespoons)*
» Eggs, large *(4)*
» Greek yogurt, nonfat plain *(15 ounces)*
» Kefir, nonfat plain *(24 ounces)*
» Milk, nonfat *(20 ounces)*
» Ricotta, part skim *(3 cups)*

MEAT

» Ham, or bacon, uncured, no nitrates added *(2 ounces; optional)*

PANTRY

DRIED HERBS AND SPICES

» Basil *(optional)*
» Black pepper, freshly ground
» Cinnamon, ground
» Dill *(optional)*
» Garlic powder
» Onion powder
» Salt

BOTTLED, CANNED, AND JARRED

» Almond butter, creamy, no added sugar
» Beans, refried, fat-free *(1 [15-ounce] can)*
» Chicken, low sodium *(1 [16-ounce] can)*
» Cooking spray, nonstick
» Marinara sauce *(1 [14-ounce] jar)*
» Mayonnaise, light
» Mustard, Dijon
» Pesto, basil
» Pico de gallo or salsa
» Tuna *(2 [3-ounce] cans)*

OTHER

» Protein shakes, commercial, with at least 15 to 30 grams of protein *(14)*

Week 2 Meal Plan: Soft Diet

	BREAKFAST	SNACK	LUNCH	SNACK	DINNER	SNACK
MONDAY	Soft Scrambled Eggs with Ricotta (page 75)	Commercial protein shake	Cheesy Cauliflower Casserole (page 77; *freeze 1 serving for another use*)	Commercial protein shake	Soft Chicken Casserole (page 82)	8 ounces nonfat kefir
TUESDAY	Banana Cottage Cheese Split (page 74)	Commercial protein shake	*Leftover* Cheesy Cauliflower Casserole	Commercial protein shake	*Leftover* Soft Chicken Casserole	5 ounces nonfat plain Greek yogurt
WEDNESDAY	Beans and Cheese with Avocado (page 79, *double the recipe*)	Commercial protein shake	*Leftover* Soft Chicken Casserole	Commercial protein shake	Ground Chicken and Cauliflower Mash (page 85)	8 ounces nonfat milk
THURSDAY	*Leftover* Beans and Cheese with Avocado	Commercial protein shake	Quick Chicken Bake (page 83)	Commercial protein shake	*Leftover* Ground Chicken and Cauliflower Mash	8 ounces nonfat kefir
FRIDAY	Baked Ricotta and Banana with Nut Butter (page 73, *double the recipe*)	Commercial protein shake	*Leftover* Quick Chicken Bake	Commercial protein shake	Meat and Potato Salad (page 86)	5 ounces nonfat plain Greek yogurt
SATURDAY	*Leftover* Baked Ricotta and Banana with Nut Butter	Commercial protein shake	*Leftover* Quick Chicken Bake	Commercial protein shake	*Leftover* Meat and Potato Salad	8 ounces nonfat milk
SUNDAY	*Leftover* Meat and Potato Salad	Commercial protein shake	*Leftover* Quick Chicken Bake	Commercial protein shake	Creamy Salmon and Dill Salad (page 81)	8 ounces nonfat kefir

Week 2 Grocery List: Soft Diet

PRODUCE

» Avocado *(1)*
» Bananas, small *(2)*
» Bell pepper, red, orange, or yellow *(1)*
» Carrot *(1)*
» Cauliflower *(2 heads)*
» Dill *(1 small container)*
» Garlic *(1 small head)*
» Lemon *(1)*
» Onion, large *(1)*
» Onion, white *(1)*
» Potatoes, russet *(3)*
» Scallions *(1 bunch)*, or chives *(1 small bunch)*
» Tomato *(1)*

FROZEN FOODS

» Hash browns, frozen *(1 cup)*

DAIRY, NONDAIRY ALTERNATIVES, AND EGGS

» Cheese, Cheddar, low fat, shredded *(1 cup)*
» Cheese, cottage, nonfat, no salt added *(¼ cup)*
» Cheese, mozzarella, low fat, shredded *(¼ cup)*
» Eggs, large *(6)*
» Greek yogurt, nonfat plain *(3 [5-ounce] containers)*
» Kefir, nonfat plain *(24 ounces)*
» Milk, nonfat *(1 quart)*
» Ricotta, part skim *(1¼ cups)*

MEAT

» Chicken, lean ground *(12 ounces)*
» Ham, cooked, no nitrates added *(4 ounces)*

PANTRY

DRIED HERBS AND SPICES

» Black pepper, freshly ground
» Cinnamon, ground
» Dill
» Garlic powder
» Salt

JARRED, BOTTLED, AND CANNED

» Almond butter, creamy, no added sugar
» Beans, refried, fat-free *(1 [15-ounce] can)*
» Chicken *(1 6-ounce] can)*
» Cooking spray, nonstick
» Jam, strawberry, sugar-free
» Mayonnaise, light
» Mustard, Dijon
» Oil, olive
» Salmon *(1 [5-ounce] can)*
» Tomatoes, diced *(1 [14.5-ounce] can)*

OTHER

» Protein shakes, commercial, with at least 15 to 30 grams of protein *(14)*

By this stage, your stomach should be healed, and you can start to introduce regular foods into your meals. The meal plans in this stage are intended to help you transition to a life of healthy eating. You can repeat these plans as many times as you'd like or start to build your own with the recipes from part 3, using the structure I provide.

During this stage, I encourage you to try new foods regularly but not to introduce several new foods at the same time to allow time to test and determine which foods you tolerate best. You may want to continue tracking your intake in your food journal to make sure you are getting enough protein and keep track of how you respond to certain foods. For the first few months, you can continue to drink commercial protein shakes between meals as a snack, if desired, to ensure that you're getting proper protein nutrition.

The main thing here is always to eat your protein first; then you can add vegetables, fruits, and healthy carbs, such as grains and starchy vegetables, and good sources of dairy. Keep in mind that red meats and tough meats may be hard to tolerate for the first few months. I suggest when transitioning to solid foods that you start with dairy, eggs, soft chicken, and seafood as your proteins. If you are getting enough protein throughout the day, you can add dessert from chapter 11 into your meal plan, as in week 2 here.

Week 1 Meal Plan: Solid Foods

	BREAKFAST	SNACK	LUNCH	SNACK	DINNER	SNACK
MONDAY	Oatmeal-Pear Smoothie (page 92)	Commercial protein shake	Easy Caprese Salad (page 107) + ½ pear + 6 small crackers	8 ounces nonfat kefir	Baked Salmon and Asparagus with Basil and Tomato (page 124)	5 ounces nonfat plain Greek yogurt + ¼ cup fresh strawberries
TUESDAY	Open-Face Feta and Basil Omelet (page 96, *double the recipe*) + 1 small apple	Commercial protein shake	Easy Caprese Salad (page 107) + ¼ cup strawberries + 6 small crackers	Commercial protein shake	*Leftover* Baked Salmon and Asparagus with Basil and Tomato	5 ounces nonfat plain Greek yogurt + ½ orange
WEDNESDAY	*Leftover* Open-Face Feta and Basil Omelet + 1 small apple	Commercial protein shake	"Mayo-less" Mediterranean Tuna Salad (page 116) + 6 small crackers	1 ounce fresh mozzarella cheese + ¼ cup strawberries	Plant-Based Protein Bowl (page 110)	5 ounces nonfat plain Greek yogurt + ½ orange
THURSDAY	Greek Yogurt, Granola, and Berry Parfait (page 93)	Commercial protein shake	*Leftover* "Mayo-less" Mediterranean Tuna Salad + 6 small crackers	8 ounces nonfat kefir + ¼ cup fresh raspberries	Orange Chicken and Quinoa (page 136)	1 tablespoon almond butter + 1 small apple
FRIDAY	Egg and Avocado Toast (page 95)	Commercial protein shake	Layered Mason Jar Chicken Salad (page 129, *triple the recipe*)	5 ounces nonfat plain Greek yogurt + ¼ cup fresh raspberries	*Leftover* Orange Chicken and Quinoa	Green Kefir Smoothie (page 105)
SATURDAY	High-Protein Porridge (page 94)	Commercial protein shake	*Leftover* Layered Mason Jar Chicken Salad	Commercial protein shake	Garlic–Olive Oil Shrimp with Quinoa (page 119)	1 tablespoon almond butter + 1 small apple
SUNDAY	High-Protein Porridge (page 94)	Commercial protein shake	*Leftover* Layered Mason Jar Chicken Salad	Commercial protein shake	*Leftover* Garlic–Olive Oil Shrimp with Quinoa	1 tablespoon almond butter + 1 small apple

Week 1 Grocery List: Solid Foods

PRODUCE

» Apples *(6)*
» Asparagus *(1 bunch)*
» Avocados *(2)*
» Basil *(1 small bunch)*
» Bell pepper, red, orange, or yellow *(1)*
» Blueberries *(1 pint)*
» Cilantro *(1 bunch)*
» Cucumbers *(3)*
» Dill *(1 small container)*
» Garlic *(1 head)*
» Lemon *(2; optional)*
» Lettuce *(1 head)*
» Onion, red *(1)*
» Oranges *(2)*
» Parsley *(1 small bunch; optional)*
» Pear *(1)*
» Scallions *(1 bunch)*
» Raspberries *(1 pint)*
» Spinach *(1 ounce)*
» Strawberries *(1 pound)*
» Tomatoes *(8)*

DAIRY, NONDAIRY ALTERNATIVES, AND EGGS

» Cheese, feta, crumbled *(1½ ounces)*
» Cheese, mozzarella, fresh *(5 ounces)*
» Eggs, large *(3)*
» Greek yogurt, nonfat plain *(24 ounces)*
» Kefir, nonfat plain *(32 ounces)*
» Milk, nonfat *(½ pint)*

MEAT AND SEAFOOD

» Chicken breast, boneless, skinless *(12 ounces)*
» Salmon *(2 [2-ounce] fillets)*
» Shrimp, fresh, peeled and deveined *(4 ounces)*

PANTRY

HERBS AND SPICES

» Basil *(optional)*
» Black pepper, freshly ground
» Cinnamon, ground
» Dill *(optional)*
» Dried garlic or 1 garlic clove
» Salt
» Vanilla extract

BOTTLED, CANNED, JARRED, AND PACKAGED

» Almond butter, creamy, no added sugar
» Capers *(1 [2.25-ounce] bottle)*
» Chickpeas, low sodium *(1 [15-ounce] can)*
» Corn *(1 [7-ounce] can)*
» Crackers, whole-grain *(1 package)*
» Dates *(1 [8-ounce] package)*
» Honey
» Jam, strawberry, sugar-free
» Mustard, Dijon
» Oats, rolled

continued »

- » Oats, steel cut *(1 [24-ounce] bag)*
- » Olives, Kalamata
  (1 [5.75-ounce] jar)
- » Oil, olive
- » Oil, vegetable
- » Pecans, chopped
  (1 [2.25-ounce] bag)
- » Pesto, basil
- » Quinoa *(1 [16-ounce] bag)*

- » Raisins, no added sugar
  (1 [12-ounce] bag)
- » Syrup, sugar-free
- » Tuna, packed in oil
  (1 [5-ounce] can)
- » Vinegar, aged balsamic
- » Walnuts, chopped
  (1 [2.25-ounce] bag)

OTHER
- » Bread, whole grain *(1 loaf)*

- » Protein shakes, commercial,
  with at least 15 to 30 grams of
  protein *(10)*

Week 2 Meal Plan: Solid Foods

	BREAKFAST	SNACK	LUNCH	SNACK	DINNER	SNACK
MONDAY	Hearty Whole-Grain Breakfast Burrito (page 100, *double the recipe*)	Commercial protein shake	Chicken Apple Salad (page 128) + 6 small crackers	8 ounces nonfat kefir + ¼ cup fresh blueberries	Lemon-Pepper Chicken and Vegetables (page 138, *double the recipe*)	Juicy Peach Dessert (page 160)
TUESDAY	*Leftover* Hearty Whole-Grain Breakfast Burrito	Commercial protein shake	*Leftover* Chicken Apple Salad + 6 small crackers	5 ounces nonfat plain Greek yogurt + ½ peach	*Leftover* Lemon-Pepper Chicken and Vegetables	Crustless Apple Pie with Nut Butter (page 161, *double the recipe*)
WEDNESDAY	Baked Egg, Parm, and Spinach Cup (page 97) + 1 small peach	Commercial protein shake	Thanksgiving-Inspired Turkey Wrap (page 141)	8 ounces nonfat kefir + ¼ cup fresh blueberries	Yogurt-Dill Salmon and Baked Potato (page 125)	*Leftover* Crustless Apple Pie with Nut Butter
THURSDAY	Turkey, Cheese, and Hash Brown Mini-Bake (page 101)	Commercial protein shake	*Leftover* Lemon-Pepper Chicken and Vegetables	5 ounces nonfat plain Greek yogurt + 1 small apple	*Leftover* Yogurt-Dill Salmon and Baked Potato	Ricotta-Stuffed Strawberries (page 164)
FRIDAY	*Leftover* Turkey, Cheese, and Hash Brown Mini-Bake	Commercial protein shake	Chickpea Salad (page 106, *double the recipe*)	5 ounces nonfat plain Greek yogurt + 1 small apple	*Leftover* Lemon-Pepper Chicken and Vegetables	*Leftover* Ricotta-Stuffed Strawberries
SATURDAY	Ricotta and Spinach Frittata (page 99, *double the recipe*)	Commercial protein shake	Thanksgiving-Inspired Turkey Wrap (page 141)	¼ cup nonfat cottage cheese + ¼ cup fresh strawberries	Pesto-Parmesan Shrimp and Broccoli (page 120)	Flourless Low-Sugar Peanut Butter Bites (page 162) + ¼ cup nonfat milk
SUNDAY	*Leftover* Ricotta and Spinach Frittata	Commercial protein shake	*Leftover* Chickpea Salad	8 ounces nonfat kefir + ¼ cup fresh strawberries	*Leftover* Pesto-Parmesan Shrimp and Broccoli	*Leftover* Flourless Low-Sugar Peanut Butter Bites + ¼ cup nonfat milk

Week 2 Grocery List: Solid Foods

PRODUCE
» Apples *(5)*
» Avocados *(2)*
» Blueberries *(1 pint)*
» Broccoli *(1 head)*
» Celery *(1 bunch)*
» Cilantro *(1 small bunch)*
» Cucumbers, Persian *(2)*
» Dill *(1 small bunch)*
» Garlic *(1 head)*
» Lemons *(2)*
» Mushrooms *(1 ounce)*
» Onion *(1)*
» Parsley *(1 bunch)*
» Peaches *(3)*
» Potato, russet *(1)*
» Scallions *(2)* or chives *(1 small bunch)*
» Spinach *(1 [5-ounce] bag)*
» Strawberries *(1 pound)*
» Tomatoes *(4)*

DAIRY, NONDAIRY ALTERNATIVES, AND EGGS
» Cheese, Cheddar, low fat, shredded *(¼ cup)*
» Cheese, cottage, nonfat, no salt added *(¼ cup)*
» Cheese, feta *(1 ounce)*
» Cheese, Parmesan, grated *(1 tablespoon)*
» Cheese, Parmesan, shredded *(1 tablespoon)*
» Cream cheese, light *(1 [8-ounce] package)*
» Eggs, large *(6)*
» Greek yogurt, nonfat plain *(1 [32-ounce] container)*
» Kefir, nonfat plain *(24 ounces)*
» Milk, nonfat *(½ pint)*
» Ricotta, part skim *(½ cup)*

FROZEN FOODS
» Hash browns, frozen *(1 cup)*
» Mixed vegetables, frozen *(1 [12-ounce] bag)*

MEAT AND SEAFOOD
» Chicken breast, boneless, skinless *(14 ounces)*
» Salmon *(2 [2-ounce fillets)*
» Shrimp, fresh, peeled and deveined *(4 ounces)*
» Turkey, cooked deli meat, no nitrates added *(4 ounces)*
» Turkey, lean ground *(4 ounces)*

PANTRY
HERBS AND SPICES
» Black pepper, freshly ground
» Cinnamon
» Dill
» Garlic powder
» Lemon pepper
» Salt
» Vanilla extract

- Almond butter, creamy, no added sugar
- Baking soda
- Beans, refried, fat-free *(1 [15-ounce] can)*
- Crackers, whole-grain *(1 package)*
- Cranberries dried, unsweetened *(1 [6-ounce] bag)*
- Chickpeas, low sodium *(1 [15-ounce] can)*
- Green chiles, diced *(1 [4.5-ounce] can)*
- Honey
- Oil, olive
- Oil, olive spray
- Peanut butter, creamy, no added sugar
- Pecans, whole *(1 [2.25-ounce] bag)*
- Pesto, basil
- Raisins, no added sugar
- Rice, brown *(1 [1-pound] bag)*
- Salsa *(optional)*
- Sugar, brown *(1 [1-pound] bag)*
- Syrup, sugar-free *(optional)*
- Syrup, sugar-free vanilla *(optional)*

OTHER

- Protein shakes, commercial, with at least 15 to 30 grams of protein *(7)*
- Tortillas, whole-grain 8-inch *(1 [6-count] package)*

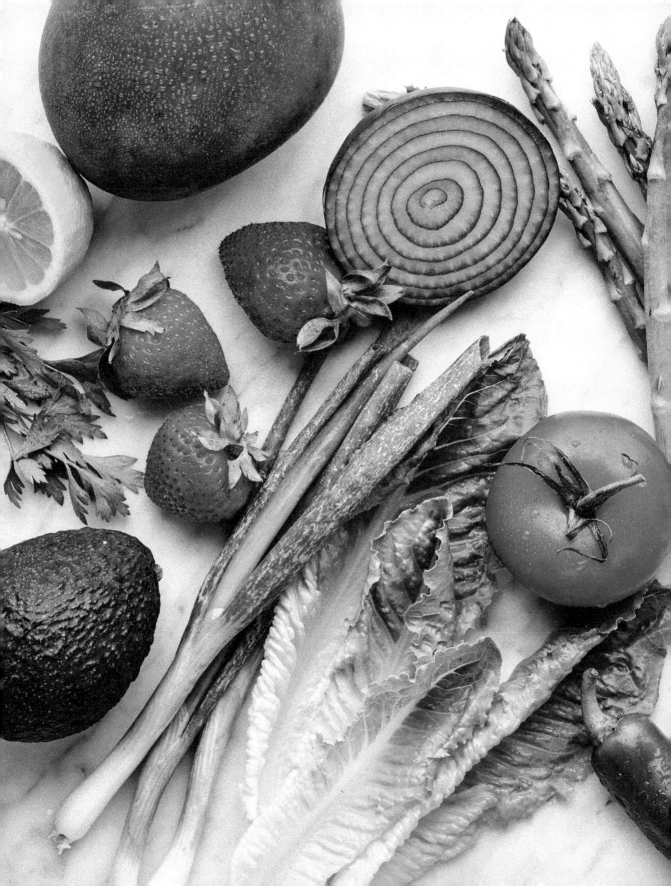

PART TWO

STAGES 1-3

RECIPES FOR RECOVERY

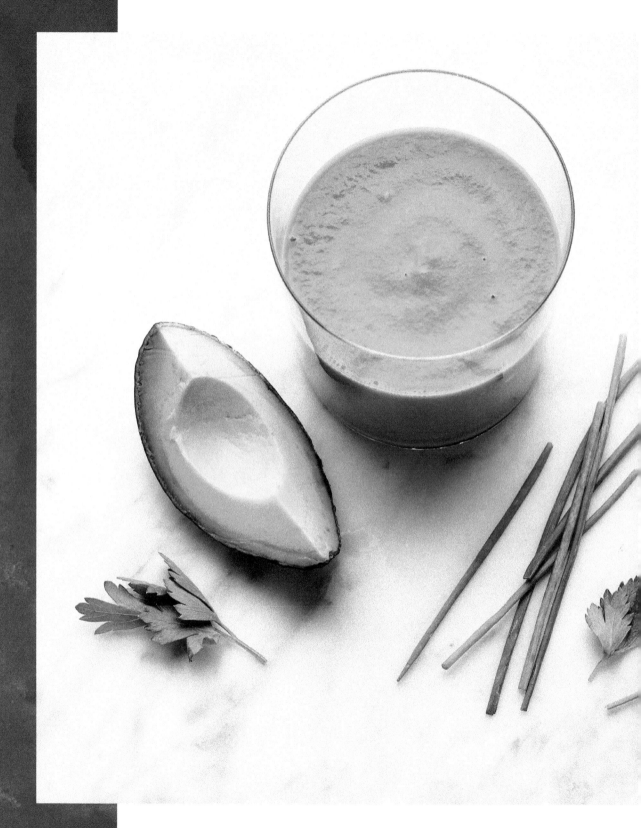

CHAPTER THREE

STAGE 1

LIQUIDS

HIGH-PROTEIN HOT CHOCOLATE MILK

5 Ingredients or Fewer
30 Minutes or Less
One Pot

SERVES 1 // **PREP TIME:** 5 minutes // **COOK TIME:** 5 minutes

Sometimes you just want a warm, comforting drink. This easy high-protein hot chocolate is made with dry milk powder, but you could use chocolate whey protein powder. You can also play around with a variety of flavored creamers, like hazelnut or coconut. I suggest using the Fairlife brand of nonfat milk, which has 13 grams of protein (compared to the usual 8 grams in other brands), less sugar, no lactose, and more calcium per serving.

1 cup nonfat milk

⅓ cup water

3 tablespoons dry milk powder

1 tablespoon unsweet-ened cacao powder

1 teaspoon sugar-free syrup or sugar-free sweetener

1 tablespoon vanilla creamer (optional)

1. In a small saucepan over medium heat, combine the milk, water, milk powder, cacao powder, and syrup. Cook for about 3 minutes to warm, stirring constantly; then remove from heat.

2. Stir in the creamer (if using), pour into a mug, and enjoy.

POST-OP TIP: Although this recipe is made with dry milk powder, it still contains milk sugar and may not be suitable for patients with lactose intolerance unless a lactase enzyme is taken before consuming.

STORAGE TIP: You can refrigerate this drink for up to 2 days in an airtight glass container. Reheat or enjoy cold.

PER SERVING *(11 ounces)*: Protein: 19g; Calories: 141; Fat: 1g; Carbohydrates: 15g; Fiber: 2g; Total sugar: 13g; Added sugar: 0g; Sodium: 190mg

NUT BUTTER ICE POPS

MAKES 8 // PREP TIME: 10 minutes, plus 6 hours or overnight to chill

5 Ingredients or Fewer
No Cook
One Pot

These ice pops are a wonderful post-surgery treat for bariatric patients because they melt in the mouth and force you to eat slowly. What's more, they freeze well for up to 3 months, so you can make a batch and enjoy one whenever you want a refreshing, protein-packed snack. For this recipe, I suggest choosing Greek yogurt or any yogurt high in protein and low in sugar and a creamy nut butter like almond or peanut butter.

2 bananas, peeled

1 cup nonfat plain Greek yogurt

½ cup creamy almond butter

1 tablespoon honey

1. In a food processor or blender, combine the bananas, yogurt, almond butter, and honey. Process until very smooth.

2. Using a rubber spatula, scrape the mixture into 8 ice pop molds and insert an ice pop stick into each mold.

3. Freeze for at least 6 hours or overnight before enjoying.

COOKING TIP: Add 1 teaspoon of a flavoring extract, such as coconut or nutmeg, for extra flavor. If you don't have ice pop molds, pour the mixture into ice-cube trays or small glass containers—roughly 2 ounces per pop.

PER SERVING (1 ice pop/2 ounces): Protein: 7g; Calories: 154; Fat: 9g; Carbohydrates: 13g; Fiber: 2g; Total sugar: 8g; Added sugar: 2g; Sodium: 12mg

CREAMY CHOCOLATE SHAKE

5 Ingredients or Fewer
30 Minutes or Less
No Cook
One Pot

SERVES 1 // **PREP TIME:** 10 minutes

If you're tired of plain protein drinks, make this creamy chocolate shake for a boost of energy. A great alternative to chocolate milk, this shake is thin, easy to drink, and low in caffeine; has no added sugar; and is rich in healthy fats from the almond butter. To change it up, add a variety of flavors, such as almond extract or maple extract; if you want this extra cold, add ice cubes before blending. I suggest using the Fairlife brand of nonfat milk, which has 13 grams of protein (compared to the usual 8 grams in other brands), less sugar, no lactose, and more calcium per serving.

8 ounces nonfat milk

1 tablespoon unsweet-ened cacao powder

1 tablespoon almond butter

1 teaspoon sugar-free vanilla syrup

½ teaspoon coconut extract (optional)

1. In a blender, combine the milk, cacao powder, almond butter, syrup, and coconut extract (if using).

2. Blend until smooth. Pour into a glass and enjoy.

3. If you prefer this beverage chilled, refrigerate for 5 to 10 minutes before sipping.

POST-OP TIP: Drink slowly, taking little sips, and do not use a straw. It may take you 30 to 40 minutes to drink one serving of this shake during the liquid stage.

COOKING TIP: If you don't want to use cow's milk, sub-stitute almond milk, coconut milk, or soy milk and 1 scoop unflavored protein powder. You may also add 1 tablespoon of half-and-half or flavored creamer for more creaminess.

PER SERVING *(9 ounces)*: Protein: 17g; Calories: 191; Fat: 10g; Carbohydrates: 11g; Fiber: 4g; Total sugar: 7g; Added sugar: 0g; Sodium: 137mg

CINNAMON-VANILLA KEFIR SHAKE

SERVES 1 // **PREP TIME:** 10 minutes

5 Ingredients or Fewer
30 Minutes or Less
No Cook
One Pot

Kefir is a tangy fermented drink with the consistency of drinkable yogurt. It is a great source of protein, vitamins, minerals, and calcium and rich in probiotics, which can aid digestive health and immune function. It is also suitable for most lactose-intolerant patients. Kefir is typically made from cow's milk and can be found in the dairy aisle at most grocery stores, but there are plenty of nondairy options available.

8 ounces nonfat plain kefir

1 tablespoon almond butter

1 teaspoon sugar-free syrup or sugar-free sweetener

½ teaspoon vanilla extract

½ teaspoon ground cinnamon

1. In a blender, combine the kefir, almond butter, syrup to taste, vanilla, and cinnamon.

2. Blend until smooth. Pour into a glass and enjoy.

COOKING TIP: You may also add ½ banana (fresh or frozen). Here is how you can freeze bananas quickly: Cut bananas into ¼- or ½-inch slices and place them on a wax paper–lined baking sheet, spaced out. Freeze for 2 hours or until solid; then transfer the frozen banana slices to a freezer-safe plastic zip-top bag or glass container. Keep frozen until needed.

PER SERVING *(9 ounces)*: Protein: 12g; Calories: 198; Fat: 11g; Carbohydrates: 14g; Fiber: 2g; Total sugar: 11g; Added sugar: 0g; Sodium: 92mg

SOY CHOCOLATE MILK SHAKE

SERVES 1 // **PREP TIME:** 10 minutes

5 Ingredients or Fewer
30 Minutes or Less
No Cook
One Pot

Soy milk contains antioxidants and isoflavones that can be beneficial against certain chronic diseases. Compared with other plant-based milk alternatives, soy milk has as much protein as cow's milk, is low in fat, and has no sugar—making it perfect for the liquid diet. This milk shake can be made with a variety of sugar-free ice cream flavors, such as caramel or chocolate. Don't have ice cream? Make Nut Butter Ice Pops (page 49) and use those as the base instead. Just defrost for 7 to 10 minutes before adding to the blender.

1 teaspoon sugar-free chocolate syrup

4 ounces sugar-free vanilla ice cream

8 ounces soy milk

1. Using a spoon, drizzle the chocolate syrup around the inside rim of a small glass.

2. In a blender, combine the ice cream and soy milk. Blend until smooth. Pour into the syrup-rimmed glass and enjoy.

POST-OP TIP: If you can't tolerate cow's milk and need a lactose-free option, use a nondairy sugar-free ice cream as your base.

PER SERVING *(12 ounces)*: Protein: 13g; Calories: 208; Fat: 4g; Carbohydrates: 35g; Fiber: 6g; Total sugar: 7g; Added sugar: 0g; Sodium: 172mg

TRIPLE ALMOND SHAKE

SERVES 1 // **PREP TIME**: 10 minutes

5 Ingredients or Fewer
30 Minutes or Less
No Cook
One Pot

This shake is dairy-free and packed with protein. Almond powder, also known as almond flour, is available in the baking or gluten-free aisles of most grocery stores. Almond flour is typically made from blanched almonds with the skins removed and is ground more finely than almond meal. The shake texture is a bit grainy, but that is normal for a vegan shake. For flavor variations, add ½ teaspoon of coconut extract or nutmeg extract.

8 ounces unsweetened almond milk

3 tablespoons almond powder

1 tablespoon almond butter

1 teaspoon sugar-free vanilla syrup

1. In a blender, combine the almond milk, almond powder, almond butter, and syrup.

2. Blend until smooth. Pour into a glass and enjoy.

COOKING TIP: For more protein, add 1 scoop of unflavored protein powder. Chocolate or vanilla protein powder is great in this shake. When you can tolerate more volume, add ½ banana (fresh or frozen) for flavor and creaminess.

PER SERVING *(9 ounces)*: Protein: 9g; Calories: 252; Fat: 22g; Carbohydrates: 8g; Fiber: 4g; Total sugar: 2g; Added sugar: 0g; Sodium: 174mg

BANANA YOGURT SHAKE

SERVES 1 // **PREP TIME**: 10 minutes

This is a refreshing snack or breakfast option when you are in a hurry and need something fast. Yogurt and banana make this shake creamy and delicious, but be sure the ingredients are fully blended. If you feel like you want to chew something, pour the shake into an ice-cube tray and freeze it into cubes. Then blend the cubes to make a slushy. Substitute soy milk for almond milk if you prefer.

½ banana, frozen

½ cup nonfat plain Greek yogurt

4 ounces unsweetened almond milk

½ teaspoon vanilla extract (optional)

1. In a blender, combine the banana, yogurt, almond milk, and vanilla (if using).

2. Blend until smooth. Pour into a glass and enjoy.

COOKING TIP: For added protein and volume, add 1 tablespoon of nut butter. You can also add unflavored, vanilla, or chocolate protein powder or swap vanilla extract (if using) for any extract flavor of choice.

PER SERVING *(9 ounces)*: Protein: 14g; Calories: 143; Fat: 2g; Carbohydrates: 19g; Fiber: 2g; Total sugar: 11; Added sugar: 0g; Sodium: 130mg

TOMATO-AVOCADO JUICE

SERVES 1 // **PREP TIME:** 10 minutes

5 Ingredients or Fewer
30 Minutes or Less
No Cook
One Pot

Although it may be easy to get enough protein in the early days of recovery, it can be difficult to get enough healthy fats. This juice is a savory way to get them into your body. If you need more protein for the day, add unflavored protein powder as needed.

8 ounces low-sodium tomato juice

¼ avocado, peeled and pitted

Salt

1 teaspoon chopped fresh parsley

¼ teaspoon chopped fresh chives (optional)

1. In a food processor or blender, combine the tomato juice and avocado. Season with salt to taste and process until very smooth.

2. Pour into a glass, garnish with parsley and chives (if using), sip, and enjoy.

STORAGE TIP: Freeze the leftover avocado to use later. Cut it into cubes or slices and brush each with a bit of freshly squeezed lemon juice. Tightly wrap the avocado in plastic wrap, leaving no room for air. Place the plastic-wrapped avocado in a freezer-safe plastic zip-top bag, tightly sealed with as much air as possible pressed out, and keep frozen until needed.

PER SERVING *(9 ounces)*: Protein: 3g; Calories: 99; Fat: 6g; Carbohydrates: 12g; Fiber: 3g; Total sugar: 6g; Added sugar: 0g; Sodium: 28mg

EASY BUTTERNUT SQUASH SOUP

SERVES 4 // **PREP TIME**: 10 minutes // **COOK TIME**: 20 minutes

Not only is this soup easy, but it can also be made sweet or savory depending on your palate preference. If you don't want to buy fresh butternut squash to peel and chop, use frozen (peeled, chopped, or riced) butternut squash as I've done here.

1 tablespoon olive oil

10 ounces frozen butternut squash

1½ cups low-sodium chicken broth

Salt

Freshly ground black pepper

2 tablespoons nonfat plain Greek yogurt, divided

2 tablespoons chopped fresh parsley, divided

1. In a medium saucepan over medium heat, combine the oil, butternut squash, and chicken broth and bring to a boil. Cook for about 10 minutes, or until the squash is very soft.

2. Remove the pan from the heat and pour the contents into a blender. Carefully blend the soup until smooth. If the soup is not thin enough, add hot water in small increments until you have the right consistency. Season with salt and pepper to taste.

3. Pour into a cup or bowl, top each serving with 1½ teaspoons of Greek yogurt, garnish with parsley, and enjoy.

STORAGE TIP: Refrigerate any remaining soup in a sealed container for up to 3 days and reheat when ready to eat. Or pour the soup into a freezer-safe glass container or plastic zip-top bag, tightly sealed with as much air as possible pressed out, and freeze for up to 6 months.

COOKING TIP: For a savory variation, add ½ teaspoon of ground cumin, dried onion, or dried garlic to taste when you season with salt and pepper. For a sweeter option, add ½ teaspoon of maple syrup or sugar-free syrup and sprinkle ground cinnamon and nutmeg to taste.

PER SERVING (5½ ounces): Protein: 2g; Calories: 71; Fat: 4g; Carbohydrates: 9g; Fiber: 2g; Total sugar: 2; Added sugar: 0g; Sodium: 50mg

CARROT-GINGER SOUP

5 Ingredients or Fewer
30 Minutes or Less

SERVES 4 // **PREP TIME:** 10 minutes // **COOK TIME:** 15 minutes

This soup is full of beta-carotene and vitamin A, thanks to the carrots, and the ginger and orange zest give it a spicy, vibrant flavor. You can change up the flavors, adding different spices, like turmeric or garlic powder, or trying a different garnish, such as chopped chives or scallion. Use fresh carrots, if you prefer; just peel and chop into small pieces.

1 tablespoon olive oil

10 ounces frozen carrots

1 tablespoon minced peeled fresh or frozen ginger

1½ cups low-sodium chicken broth or vegetable broth

3 large strips orange peel

Salt

Freshly ground black pepper

4 teaspoons nonfat plain Greek yogurt, divided

Chopped fresh parsley, for garnish (optional)

1. In a medium saucepan over medium heat, combine the oil, carrots, ginger, chicken broth, and orange peel. Bring the soup to a boil and cook for 10 to 15 minutes until the carrots are very soft. Remove from the heat. Remove and discard the orange peel.

2. Carefully pour the soup into a blender and blend on high speed until smooth. Season with salt and pepper to taste.

3. Serve in glasses or bowls and top each serving with 1 teaspoon of Greek yogurt and a sprinkle of fresh parsley (if using) to enjoy.

STORAGE TIP: Refrigerate leftover soup in an airtight container for up to 3 days and reheat when ready to eat. Or, freeze it in an airtight container or freezer-safe plastic zip-top bag, tightly sealed with as much air as possible pressed out, for up to 6 months.

PER SERVING *(5½ ounces)*: Protein: 2g; Calories: 76; Fat: 4g; Carbohydrates: 9g; Fiber: 3g; Total sugar: 5g; Added sugar: 0g; Sodium: 94mg

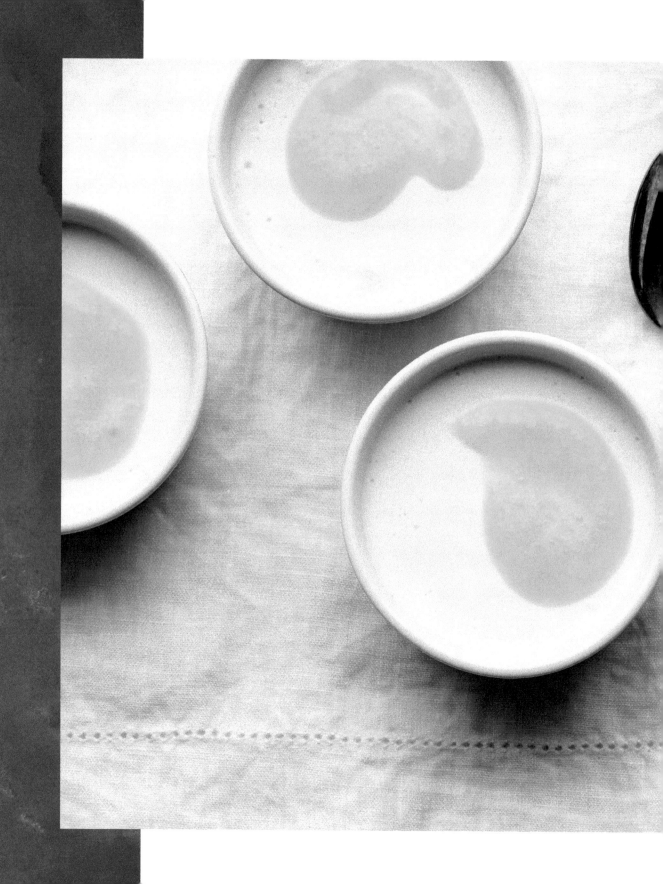

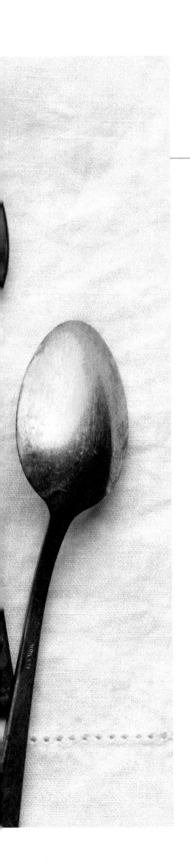

CHAPTER FOUR

STAGE 2

PUREES

HERB AND MELON KEFIR SMOOTHIE

30 Minutes or Less
No Cook
One Pot

SERVES 1 // **PREP TIME:** 10 minutes

This smoothie is a beautiful blend of fresh herbs and melon, and it provides protein, probiotics, fiber, and antioxidants—all beneficial to your post-op health. It's also a great way to start adding fruits into your diet. With its fresh taste, this smoothie is great for those who do not like very sweet drinks. For variety or taste preference, swap the honeydew for cantaloupe, substitute buttermilk for kefir, and use fresh or frozen herbs.

4 ounces nonfat plain kefir

¼ cup nonfat plain Greek yogurt

¾ cup chopped honeydew melon

4 fresh mint leaves

2 fresh basil leaves

1 teaspoon honey

¼ teaspoon vanilla extract

1. In a blender, combine the kefir, yogurt, melon, mint, basil, honey, and vanilla.

2. Blend until smooth, or until your desired consistency is reached. Pour into a glass and enjoy.

PER SERVING *(12 ounces)*: Protein: 11g; Calories: 159; Fat: 2g; Carbohydrates: 26g; Fiber: 1g; Total sugar: 25g; Added sugar: 6g; Sodium: 94mg

KEFIR AND YOGURT BANANA FLAXSEED SHAKE

5 Ingredients or Fewer
30 Minutes or Less
No Cook
One Pot

SERVES 1 // **PREP TIME**: 10 minutes, plus 15 minutes to chill

This shake is full of protein, vitamins, minerals, calcium, and probiotics. You can find sunflower seed butter in the nut butter section of most grocery stores or swap it for your favorite nut butter. This drink is best enjoyed chilled, but you can skip that step if desired or simply blend in two or three ice cubes.

⅓ cup nonfat plain kefir

6 ounces nonfat plain Greek yogurt

½ banana, fresh or frozen

1 tablespoon ground flaxseed

1 tablespoon sunflower seed butter

1 teaspoon sugar-free vanilla syrup or honey (optional)

1. In a blender, combine the kefir, yogurt, banana, flaxseed, sunflower seed butter, and syrup (if using).

2. Blend until smooth. Pour into a glass and enjoy.

3. Alternatively, refrigerate for 10 to 15 minutes to chill before sipping.

POST-OP TIP: This recipe is helpful for someone who suffers from constipation. Constipation is common after surgery due to low fiber intake from fruits, vegetable, and grains. Ground flaxseed, high in omega-3 fatty acids, is a great addition to any yogurt or smoothie and even soups to help get things moving.

PER SERVING *(12 ounces)*: Protein: 26g; Calories: 329; Fat: 14g; Carbohydrates: 28g; Fiber: 5g; Total sugar: 17g; Added sugar: 0g; Sodium: 157mg

PIÑA COLADA SMOOTHIE

SERVES 1 // **PREP TIME**: 10 minutes, plus up to 15 minutes to chill

5 Ingredients or Fewer
30 Minutes or Less
No Cook
One Pot

This refreshing smoothie, with its tropical flavors of pineapple and coconut, will make you feel like you're sitting on a sunny beach. I suggest using canned pineapple with no added sugar, or packed in light syrup. In some stores, you can find low-sugar vanilla or coconut Greek yogurt, which makes this smoothie even better.

½ cup canned pineapple chunks, drained

4 ounces unsweetened coconut milk

½ cup nonfat plain Greek yogurt

½ teaspoon coconut extract

1. In a blender, combine the pineapple, coconut milk, yogurt, and coconut extract.

2. Blend until smooth, or until your desired consistency is reached. Pour into a glass and enjoy.

3. Alternatively, refrigerate for 10 to 15 minutes to chill before sipping.

POST-OP TIP: Drink smoothies slowly, a few sips at a time, to get your fruits in during the day. Refrigerate what you do not finish and come back to it later. When you are in Stage 4 and beyond, add 1 tablespoon of dried shredded coconut to enhance the taste.

PER SERVING *(12 ounces)*: Protein: 13g; Calories: 148; Fat: 3g; Carbohydrates: 19g; Fiber: 1g; Total sugar: 17g; Added sugar: 0g; Sodium: 46mg

GREEN MANGO SMOOTHIE

SERVES 1 // **PREP TIME:** 10 minutes

30 Minutes or Less
No Cook
One Pot

A lot of my patients miss eating fruits and vegetables. As you progress through the pureed diet, you can start making a variety of smoothies, which is an easy way to enjoy these foods and nourish your body. Be sure not to add too much fruit—use more vegetables in your smoothies for less sugar and fewer calories. In this recipe, you can substitute canned pineapple for the mango. I suggest choosing canned fruits with no added sugar or that are packed in light syrup.

⅓ avocado, peeled and pitted

⅓ cup fresh spinach

½ cup canned mango chunks, drained

½ cup nonfat plain Greek yogurt

½ cup nonfat milk

1 teaspoon honey or sugar-free vanilla syrup

1. In a blender, combine the avocado, spinach, mango, yogurt, milk, and honey.

2. Blend until smooth, or until your desired consistency is reached. Pour into a glass and enjoy.

POST-OP TIP: Drink smoothies slowly, a few sips at a time. Refrigerate what you do not finish and come back to it later. As you progress with your diet, make this smoothie with fresh or frozen mango or pineapple.

PER SERVING *(12 ounces)*: Protein: 21g; Calories: 261; Fat: 8g; Carbohydrates: 30g; Fiber: 5g; Total sugar: 24g; Added sugar: 6g; Sodium: 117mg

PEACHY GREEK YOGURT PANNA COTTA

SERVES 4 // **PREP TIME:** 10 minutes // **COOK TIME:** 10 minutes, plus 2 to 8 hours to chill

This recipe is one of my favorites, and I am excited to share it with you. Once you advance to a solid foods diet, canned fruit can be swapped for any kind of fresh or frozen fruit—berries work great. This recipe is even better with 2% yogurt. You can also use sugar-free syrup instead of honey to lower your sugar intake.

½ cup nonfat milk

1½ tablespoons honey

1 tablespoon unflavored powdered gelatin

1½ cups nonfat plain Greek yogurt

½ teaspoon vanilla extract (optional)

½ cup canned no-sugar-added sliced peaches, drained

1. In a small saucepan over low heat, heat the milk for 2 to 4 minutes until lukewarm. Add the honey and gelatin. Cook for 3 to 5 minutes, stirring, until the honey and gelatin dissolve. (Do not bring to a boil.) Remove from the heat.

2. In a small bowl, whisk the yogurt until smooth. Add the warm gelatin mixture and vanilla (if using). Whisk well to combine. Pour into 4 small jars, glasses, or ramekins. Refrigerate for at least 2 hours or overnight for best results.

3. Before serving, put the canned peaches into a blender or food processor and puree until smooth.

4. Top each panna cotta with 2 tablespoons of pureed peach and enjoy.

STORAGE TIP: Refrigerate leftover panna cotta, in covered glass containers or ramekins, for up to 5 days.

COOKING TIP: If you don't have time to make panna cotta, you can enjoy the same flavors simply by spooning ½ cup of yogurt into a small jar, glass, or ramekin and topping with pureed fruit.

PER SERVING *(5 ounces)*: Protein: 12g; Calories: 106; Fat: 1g; Carbohydrates: 13g; Fiber: <1g; Total sugar: 13g; Added sugar: 7g; Sodium: 48mg

NUTTY CREAMY WHEAT BOWL

5 Ingredients or Fewer
30 Minutes or Less
One Pot

SERVES 1 // **PREP TIME**: 5 minutes // **COOK TIME**: 10 minutes

Cream of Wheat is a popular option for people on a pureed diet. To add more protein to this recipe, I use milk and almond butter instead of regular butter. (I recommend using Fairlife milk as it has more protein per serving than others.) Breakfast cereal just got better—and healthier.

4 ounces nonfat milk

1 tablespoon uncooked Cream of Wheat

Salt

1 teaspoon almond butter

Ground cinnamon, for seasoning

½ banana, mashed

1. In a small saucepan or pot, stir together the milk and Cream of Wheat until combined. Place the pot over medium-high heat and bring the mixture to a boil, whisking frequently to keep lumps from forming.

2. Reduce the heat to low and simmer the cereal for 1 to 2 minutes, just until it thickens. Season with salt to taste and pour the cereal into a bowl.

3. Add the almond butter and season with cinnamon. Top the cereal with mashed banana before enjoying.

POST-OP TIP: Eat slowly, one bite at a time. You don't have to finish the whole portion. Eat the cereal with nut butter first, and if you can eat more, finish the fruit.

PER SERVING *(5 ounces)*: Protein: 10; Calories: 167; Fat: 3g; Carbohydrates: 26g; Fiber: 2g; Total sugar: 11g; Added sugar: 0g; Sodium: 127mg

BAKED CINNAMON-APPLE RICOTTA

5 Ingredients or Fewer
30 Minutes or Less
One Pot

SERVES 1 // **PREP TIME**: 10 minutes // **COOK TIME**: 15 minutes

This simple recipe is great for breakfast or lunch—or dessert. It is very smooth and can be easily tolerated when you start incorporating pureed foods into your meals, and in combination with ricotta, it has a creamy mouthfeel. Plus, applesauce has vitamin C, which is beneficial for immune function.

½ cup part-skim ricotta

¼ cup no-sugar-added applesauce

1 teaspoon ground cinnamon

Ground nutmeg, for seasoning (optional)

1. Preheat the oven to 375°F.

2. Spoon the ricotta into a 6-ounce ramekin. Top with the applesauce and sprinkle with the cinnamon and nutmeg (if using) to taste.

3. Bake for 15 minutes, or until hot. Remove and let cool slightly before enjoying warm.

STORAGE TIP: Double or triple this recipe, let cool, and then refrigerate, covered, for up to 3 days. Reheat when ready to eat.

PER SERVING *(5½ ounces)*: Protein: 14g; Calories: 202; Fat: 10g; Carbohydrates:15g; Fiber: 2g; Total sugar: 6g; Added sugar: 0g; Sodium: 123mg

DECADENT TOMATO-BASIL SOUP

SERVES 4 // **PREP TIME:** 10 minutes // **COOK TIME:** 20 minutes

This soup is full of lycopene, a powerful phytonutrient found in processed tomatoes and full of health benefits, including for heart health and cancer prevention. This soup is a great savory option for your recovery and, thanks to its many health benefits, should be included in your lifestyle regimen. On the pureed diet, try the recipe as written. When you fully recover, pair it with Parmesan Crisps (page 170) or sourdough toast, and top with 1 tablespoon of Sundried Tomato Pesto (page 169).

2 tablespoons olive oil

¼ cup diced purple onion

1 (15-ounce) can low-sodium whole tomatoes or diced tomatoes, with their juices

8 ounces low-sodium chicken broth or vegetable broth

1 teaspoon dried basil

2 teaspoons honey

1 teaspoon aged balsamic vinegar (optional)

Salt

Freshly ground black pepper

8 tablespoons nonfat plain Greek yogurt

1. In a medium saucepan over medium heat, heat the oil. Add the onion and sauté for about 5 minutes until golden.

2. Stir in the tomatoes with their juices, chicken broth, and basil and bring the soup to a boil. Reduce the heat to low, cover the pan, and simmer the soup for 10 to 15 minutes. Remove from the heat.

3. Carefully pour the soup into a blender and blend on high speed until smooth. Add the honey and vinegar (if using). Season with salt and pepper to taste. Pour into glasses or bowls. Top each serving with 2 tablespoons of yogurt for extra protein and enjoy.

STORAGE TIP: Refrigerate leftover soup in an airtight container for up to 3 days and reheat when ready to eat. Top with yogurt after reheating.

COOKING TIP: Instead of basil, use oregano or a mix of both. Instead of honey, use agave syrup, and instead of black pepper try cayenne pepper to taste if you like things spicy.

PER SERVING *(5½ ounces)*: Protein: 4g; Calories: 121; Fat: 7g; Carbohydrates: 9g; Fiber: 1g; Total sugar: 7g; Added sugar: 3g; Sodium: 164mg

EASY GREEN PEA AND HAM SOUP

5 Ingredients or Fewer
30 Minutes or Less

SERVES 5 // **PREP TIME:** 10 minutes // **COOK TIME:** 20 minutes

If you like peas and ham, you will love this recipe. It is very easy to make, tastes great, and smells so good. Use frozen green peas to make this soup, and choose uncured, no-nitrates-added Canadian bacon or ham. Because ham and broth are typically salty, you probably won't need to add salt.

1 tablespoon olive oil

1 (10-ounce) package frozen peas

4 ounces ham or Canadian bacon, cut into ¼-inch cubes

1½ cups low-sodium chicken broth or vegetable broth

⅓ cup nonfat plain Greek yogurt

Freshly ground black pepper

Chopped fresh parsley, for garnish

1. In a medium saucepan over medium-high heat, heat the oil.

2. Add the peas, ham, and chicken broth and bring to a boil. Cook for about 10 minutes, or until the peas are very soft. Remove from the heat.

3. Carefully pour the soup into a blender and puree until smooth. Pour into bowls or cups. Top each serving with 1 tablespoon of yogurt and season with pepper to taste. Garnish with parsley and enjoy.

STORAGE TIP: Refrigerate leftover soup in an airtight container for up to 3 days and reheat when ready to eat. Or freeze in an airtight glass container or freezer-safe plastic zip-top bag, tightly sealed with as much air as possible pressed out, for up to 6 months.

PER SERVING (5 ounces): Protein: 11g; Calories: 116; Fat: 4g; Carbohydrates: 9g; Fiber: 3g; Total sugar: 4g; Added sugar: 0g; Sodium: 327mg

SAVORY CHICKEN SALAD

SERVES 4 // **PREP TIME:** 10 minutes

30 Minutes or Less
No Cook

Sometimes patients crave meat after surgery, but it can be hard to tolerate meats at the beginning. Canned chicken is very soft and easier to tolerate. Typically, a small 5-ounce can of chicken contains about 3½ ounces of meat after it's been drained, whereas a large 12-ounce can has about 8 ounces. In this recipe, you can swap Greek yogurt for light mayonnaise and season with cumin or dried celery in addition to the garlic powder and onion powder if desired.

1 (12-ounce) can low-sodium canned chicken, drained (about 8 ounces)

3 tablespoons plain nonfat Greek yogurt

1 tablespoon chopped scallion or fresh chives (optional)

1 teaspoon chopped fresh dill (optional)

¼ teaspoon garlic powder

⅛ teaspoon onion powder

Salt

Freshly ground black pepper

1. Place the chicken into a food processor and blend until smooth.

2. Transfer the chicken to a medium bowl and add the yogurt, scallion (if using), dill (if using), garlic powder, and onion powder. Season with salt and pepper to taste. Mix well and enjoy.

3. Refrigerate leftovers in an airtight container for up to 3 days.

COOKING TIP: If you don't have a food processer, vigorously mash the chicken with a fork until smooth. Canned chicken is very soft and falls apart easily. You can also mix the chicken with pesto for added flavor and nutrients.

PER SERVING *(2 ounces)*: Protein: 13g; Calories: 71; Fat: 1g; Carbohydrates: 1g; Fiber: 0g; Total sugar: <1g; Added sugar: 0g; Sodium: 254mg

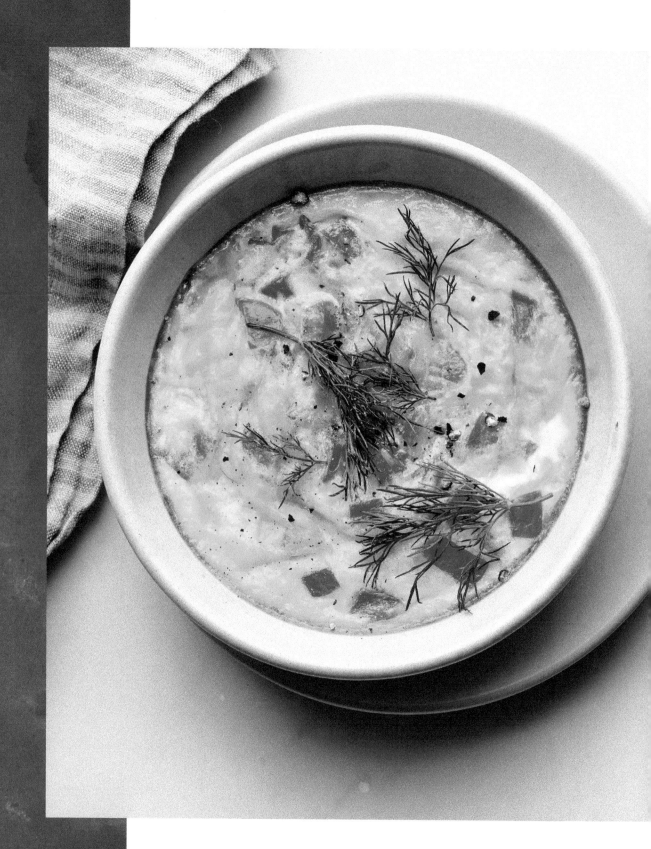

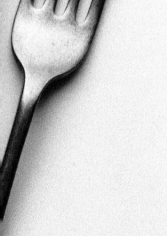

CHAPTER FIVE

STAGE 3

SOFT FOODS

RISE-AND-SHINE
BREAKFAST SOUFFLÉ

5 Ingredients or Fewer
30 Minutes or Less
One Pot

SERVES 1 // **PREP TIME:** 5 minutes // **COOK TIME:** 15 minutes

This recipe makes a soft, moist soufflé. Although you can add ham or bacon, I suggest trying this soufflé without meat first to test for tolerance and volume. If you choose to make it with ham or bacon, purchase uncured meat with no added nitrates and do not add salt. Parsley or cilantro can be substituted for dill if you prefer.

1 large egg

¼ cup nonfat milk

Salt

Freshly ground
  black pepper

1 ounce ham or bacon,
  chopped (optional)

½ tomato, diced

2 tablespoons shredded
  low-fat Cheddar cheese

Dill, fresh or dried, for
  seasoning (optional)

1. Preheat the oven to 350°F.

2. In a medium bowl, combine the egg and milk and season with salt and pepper to taste. Whisk to combine well. Whisk in the ham (if using). Pour the egg mixture into a 6-ounce ramekin. Sprinkle on the tomato, Cheddar cheese, and dill (if using).

3. Bake for 10 to 15 minutes until the egg is set and the cheese is lightly browned. Remove from the oven and let the soufflé cool slightly before enjoying warm.

STORAGE TIP: Make several portions of this soufflé and refrigerate them, covered, for up to 2 days. Reheat in the microwave when you are ready to eat.

PER SERVING *(1 ramekin; 4 ounces)*: Protein: 13g; Calories: 124; Fat: 6g; Carbohydrates: 5g; Fiber: 1g; Total sugar: 4g; Added sugar: 0g; Sodium: 211mg

BAKED RICOTTA AND BANANA WITH NUT BUTTER

5 Ingredients or Fewer
30 Minutes or Less
One Pot

SERVES 1 // **PREP TIME:** 5 minutes // **COOK TIME:** 10 minutes

This simple recipe is a great option for breakfast, lunch, dinner—or dessert. As you progress through recovery and are able to tolerate nuts instead of nut butter, add roasted nuts to this dish for crunch. For this recipe, I prefer creamy almond butter, but creamy peanut butter is equally delicious. If you don't have a banana, substitute 1 teaspoon of sugar-free jam.

½ cup part-skim ricotta

¼ cup diced banana

1 tablespoon almond butter

1 teaspoon ground cinnamon

1. Preheat the oven to 350°F.

2. In a 6-ounce ramekin, layer the ricotta, banana, and almond butter. Sprinkle with cinnamon.

3. Bake for 10 minutes, or until hot. Let cool slightly and enjoy warm.

STORAGE TIP: You can easily double or triple this recipe. Once baked, let fully cool; then refrigerate, covered, for up to 3 days. Microwave to reheat when you are ready to eat.

PER SERVING *(6 ounces)*: Protein: 18g; Calories: 306; Fat: 19g; Carbohydrates: 20g; Fiber: 4g; Total sugar: 6g; Added sugar: 0g; Sodium: 124mg

BANANA COTTAGE CHEESE SPLIT

SERVES 1 // **PREP TIME:** 5 minutes

5 Ingredients or Fewer
30 Minutes or Less
No Cook
One Pot

This combination is very appealing to the eye and tastes great, and you can make several variations. When buying cottage cheese, choose one with no salt added. Consider brands like Muuna, Good Culture, and Lifeway farmer's cheese. Try this recipe with different jam flavors, like cherry or grape, and a variety of nut butters—almond, peanut, or sunflower seed. You can also use ricotta if you prefer it to cottage cheese.

1 small banana

¼ cup nonfat cottage cheese

1 tablespoon sugar-free strawberry jam

1 tablespoon almond butter

Ground cinnamon, for seasoning (optional)

1. Halve the banana lengthwise and place it, open, on a plate.

2. Top the banana with the cottage cheese, jam, and almond butter.

3. Sprinkle with cinnamon to taste (if using). Enjoy immediately.

POST-OP TIP: This recipe is ideal for the soft diet, but as you progress and are able to eat a greater variety of foods, you can enjoy several variations. For example, add ground flaxseed, nuts, shredded coconut, or seeds such as chia, pumpkin, or sunflower. By adding these ingredients, you increase your fiber intake, which can help prevent constipation.

PER SERVING *(4 ounces)*: Protein: 11g; Calories: 251; Fat: 11g; Carbohydrates: 33g; Fiber: 4g; Total sugar: 15g; Added sugar: 0g; Sodium: 172mg

SOFT SCRAMBLED EGGS WITH RICOTTA

5 Ingredients or Fewer
30 Minutes or Less

SERVES 1 // **PREP TIME:** 5 minutes // **COOK TIME:** 10 minutes

Soft, fluffy eggs with a touch of ricotta are both nutritious and tasty. The texture is creamy but light, making this meal easy to tolerate. It takes only a few minutes to make, and the eggs and cheese provide lots of protein.

1 large egg

1 tablespoon nonfat milk

1 teaspoon chopped scallion or fresh chives

Salt

1 teaspoon olive oil or olive oil spray

2 tablespoons part-skim ricotta

1. In a small bowl, whisk the egg, milk, scallion, and salt to taste until well combined.

2. In a small skillet over medium heat, heat the oil. Add the egg mixture. Cook for about 2 minutes, stirring, until the eggs are almost cooked.

3. Stir in the ricotta just until incorporated, with clumps of cheese still visible. Remove from the heat, spoon onto a plate, and enjoy warm.

COOKING TIP: Use liquid eggs instead of fresh eggs, or add feta cheese instead of ricotta.

PER SERVING *(3 ounces)*: Protein: 10g; Calories: 144; Fat: 11g; Carbohydrates: 3g; Fiber: 0g; Total sugar: 2g; Added sugar: 0g; Sodium: 136mg

SCALLION AND MUSTARD EGG SALAD

5 Ingredients or Fewer
30 Minutes or Less
No Cook
One Pot

SERVES 2 // **PREP TIME:** 20 minutes, plus 10 minutes to chill

This simple dish is light and tasty and can be served for lunch or dinner. Eggs are tolerated by most patients, and scallions enhance flavor while providing additional health benefits: They are packed with antioxidants, provide anti-inflammatory benefits, and have antibacterial properties. If desired, enjoy with soft crackers.

2 hard-boiled eggs, peeled and diced

2 teaspoons chopped scallion or fresh chives

1 teaspoon chopped fresh dill, or ¼ teaspoon dried (optional)

1 tablespoon light mayonnaise

1½ teaspoons Dijon mustard

Salt

Freshly ground black pepper

1. In a medium bowl, combine the eggs, scallion, dill (if using), mayonnaise, and Dijon.

2. Season with salt and pepper to taste. Mix well.

3. Enjoy immediately, or chill for 10 minutes before eating.

STORAGE TIP: Double or triple this recipe and refrigerate it in an airtight container for up to 3 days.

COOKING TIP: To boil the eggs: In a small saucepan over high heat, bring 3 cups of water to a boil. Reduce the heat to low and gently add the eggs; then turn the heat to high again. Cook for 12 to 14 minutes, depending on how firm you want your egg yolks. Transfer the cooked eggs to an ice bath or run under cold water. Once the eggs are almost cool, peel. To save time, buy precooked eggs.

PER SERVING (⅓ *cup*): Protein: 6g; Calories: 90; Fat: 7 g; Carbohydrates: 1g; Fiber: <1g; Total sugar: 1g; Added sugar: 0 g; Sodium: 210mg

CHEESY CAULIFLOWER CASSEROLE

SERVES 3 // **PREP TIME:** 5 minutes // **COOK TIME:** 30 minutes

This comfort-food dish is a great way to get your vegetables while still following the soft diet guidelines. On the soft diet, it is important to eat fully cooked vegetables. This recipe is high in protein, easy to make, and simply delicious. You can use fresh garlic or pre-minced if you prefer.

1 tablespoon olive oil

1 tablespoon water

1 garlic clove, minced

1 cup diced cauliflower florets

Salt

Freshly ground black pepper

1 large egg

¼ cup nonfat plain Greek yogurt

2 tablespoons nonfat milk

¼ cup shredded low-fat Cheddar cheese

2 tablespoons chopped scallion

Fresh parsley, for garnish (optional)

1. Preheat the oven to 425°F.

2. In a medium skillet over low heat, heat the oil. Add the water, garlic, and cauliflower. Season with salt and pepper to taste. Sauté for 10 minutes, or until the cauliflower is soft.

3. Meanwhile, in a small bowl, whisk the egg, yogurt, and milk until smooth.

4. When the cauliflower is cooked, transfer it to a 9-by-5 inch glass or ceramic baking dish and pour the egg mixture over the top. Top with the Cheddar cheese and scallion; then cover the dish with aluminum foil.

5. Bake for 15 minutes. Uncover and bake for 5 minutes more until the casserole is set and the cheese is melted. Remove from the oven and top the casserole with parsley (if using). Enjoy warm.

STORAGE TIP: Refrigerate leftover casserole in an airtight container for up to 3 days, or freeze for up to 3 months.

PER SERVING *(4 ounces)*: Protein: 7g; Calories: 109; Fat: 7g; Carbohydrates: 4g; Fiber: 1g; Total sugar: 2g; Added sugar: 0g; Sodium: 123mg

RICOTTA WITH TOMATO SAUCE AND PARMESAN

5 Ingredients or Fewer
30 Minutes or Less
One Pot

SERVES 1 // **PREP TIME:** 5 minutes // **COOK TIME:** 15 minutes

This recipe is like lasagna but without the carb-heavy noodles. I love making this with a simple marinara sauce, but you can try it with any tomato-based pasta sauce you like: garlic, tomato and basil, or arrabbiata. Avoid creamy cheese-based sauces, as they are typically high in fat. This recipe tastes better if you add shredded, shaved, or freshly grated Parmesan—or omit the Parmesan for less fat and fewer calories.

½ cup part-skim ricotta

¼ cup marinara sauce

1 tablespoon dried basil (optional)

1 tablespoon shredded or shaved Parmesan cheese

1 or 2 fresh basil leaves (optional)

1. Preheat the oven to 375°F.

2. In a 6-ounce ramekin, layer the ricotta and marinara sauce. Sprinkle with the dried basil (if using). Top with the Parmesan cheese.

3. Bake for 15 minutes, or until hot and the cheese is melted.

4. Garnish with fresh basil (if using) and enjoy warm.

STORAGE TIP: Bake several ramekins of this delicious dish at one time. Once cool, tightly cover with plastic wrap and refrigerate for up to 3 days. Reheat in the microwave when ready to eat.

PER SERVING *(1 ramekin; 6 ounces)*: Protein: 13g; Calories: 181; Fat: 8g; Carbohydrates: 13g; Fiber: 1g; Total sugar: 11g; Added sugar: 0g; Sodium: 429mg

BEANS AND CHEESE WITH AVOCADO

5 Ingredients or Fewer
30 Minutes or Less
One Pot

SERVES 1 // **PREP TIME:** 5 minutes // **COOK TIME:** 5 minutes

Beans are a soft and easy source of protein and fiber. They're also inexpensive, store well in the pantry, and can be used in many ways across many types of dishes. For this recipe, I suggest purchasing canned fat-free refried beans. I also prefer using canola oil spray to avoid unnecessary added fat, but you can use 1 teaspoon of olive oil to heat the beans.

Nonstick cooking spray

¼ cup fat-free refried beans

1 tablespoon shredded low-fat Cheddar cheese

1 tablespoon pico de gallo or salsa (optional)

⅛ medium avocado, peeled, pitted, and diced (optional)

1. Coat a small skillet with cooking spray and place it over medium heat. Place the refried beans in the skillet, top with the Cheddar cheese, and cook for about 5 minutes to heat through. Remove from the heat and spoon the beans and cheese into a small bowl.

2. Top with pico de gallo (if using) and avocado (if using). Enjoy immediately.

POST-OP TIP: Try just the beans and cheese portion of this recipe and see how you feel. If you think you can add additional foods, like salsa or avocado, add a small amount and see how you tolerate it. You may increase your portion size to ½ cup of beans when you can tolerate more food. Eat slowly and stop when you feel full.

PER SERVING (3 ounces): Protein: 5g; Calories: 58; Fat: 1g; Carbohydrates: 8g; Fiber: 3g; Total sugar: <1g; Added sugar: 0g; Sodium: 263mg

TUNA-AVOCADO SALAD

SERVES 2 // **PREP TIME**: 10 minutes

5 Ingredients or Fewer
30 Minutes or Less
No Cook
One Pot

This creamy, delicious salad can be enjoyed on its own or paired with soft crackers or Parmesan Crisps (page 170). It is full of protein from the tuna and healthy fats from the avocado. Try this recipe with canned salmon, too, and swap dill for cilantro or parsley if preferred.

¼ avocado, peeled, pitted, and diced

½ teaspoon freshly squeezed lemon juice

4 ounces canned tuna, drained

1 tablespoon light mayonnaise

1 tablespoon Dijon mustard

Chopped dill, fresh or dried, for seasoning (optional)

1. In a small bowl, combine the avocado and lemon juice. Use a fork to mix well.

2. Add the tuna, mayonnaise, Dijon, and dill (if using) and mix well with a fork. Enjoy immediately.

STORAGE TIP: Refrigerate leftovers in an airtight container for up to 2 days.

POST-OP TIP: As you progress in your recovery and introduce more foods into your diet, change up this salad by adding diced sundried tomatoes and fresh onion. For some kick, add 1 teaspoon of wasabi or hot sauce.

PER SERVING *(2½ ounces)*: Protein: 15g; Calories: 120; Fat: 5g; Carbohydrates: 3g; Fiber: 1g; Total sugar: <1g; Added sugar: 0g; Sodium: 275mg

CREAMY SALMON AND DILL SALAD

30 Minutes or Less
No Cook
One Pot

SERVES 2 // **PREP TIME:** 10 minutes

Salmon is full of healthy omega-3 fatty acids. You can eat this high-protein salad with soft crackers or Parmesan Crisps (page 170) or on top of a lettuce leaf. The Dijon mustard adds flavor and creaminess without increasing fat. You can use creamy or whole-grain Dijon. You can also incorporate this salad into deviled eggs: Simply halve hard-boiled eggs lengthwise, scoop out the yolk, and put a teaspoon of this salad in its place. If you have fresh dill on hand, this recipe will taste even better.

4 ounces canned salmon, drained

2 hard-boiled eggs, peeled and chopped

2 tablespoons light mayonnaise

1 teaspoon Dijon mustard

Chopped dill, fresh or dried, for seasoning

Freshly ground black pepper

Freshly squeezed lemon juice, for seasoning

1. In a small bowl, combine the salmon, eggs, mayonnaise, and Dijon. Season with dill and pepper to taste. Add a splash of lemon juice to taste.

2. Stir well to combine and enjoy immediately.

POST-OP TIP: As you progress through recovery, add chopped fresh cucumber or diced onion to this salad. You can also make this recipe with canned tuna or canned boneless sardines if preferred.

PER SERVING *(4 ounces)*: Protein: 19g; Calories: 185; Fat: 11g; Carbohydrates: 2g; Fiber: <1g; Total sugar: 1g; Added sugar: 0g; Sodium: 460mg

SOFT CHICKEN CASSEROLE

SERVES 3 // **PREP TIME:** 5 minutes // **COOK TIME:** 25 minutes

This recipe makes a deliciously creamy, savory casserole that is perfect for lunch or dinner. It can be made with fresh boneless, skinless chicken breast, but using canned chicken ensures softness as well as reduces the cooking and preparation time. I suggest using low-sodium canned chicken.

1 tablespoon olive oil

¼ cup diced red bell pepper

¼ cup diced onion

¼ cup nonfat milk

1 large egg

Salt

Freshly ground black pepper

6 ounces low-sodium canned chicken, drained

¼ cup shredded low-fat Cheddar cheese

½ teaspoon paprika (optional)

Chopped fresh parsley, for garnish (optional)

1. Preheat the oven to 350°F.

2. In a medium skillet over low heat, heat the oil. Add the red bell pepper and onion. Sauté for about 7 minutes, stirring occasionally, until soft and the onion is golden.

3. Meanwhile, in a medium bowl, combine the milk and egg and season with salt and pepper to taste. Mix well with a fork or whisk. Add the chicken and stir well to combine. Spoon the chicken mixture into a small 9-by-5-inch glass or ceramic baking dish. Top with the sautéed vegetables and sprinkle with the Cheddar cheese. Cover the dish with aluminum foil.

4. Bake for 15 minutes. Remove the foil and bake for 3 minutes more, or until the cheese is golden brown. Serve hot with a dash of paprika (if using), garnish with parsley (if using), and enjoy.

STORAGE TIP: Let the casserole cool; then tightly cover the dish with plastic wrap or place the cooled casserole in an airtight container, and refrigerate for up to 3 days.

PER SERVING (*4 ounces*): Protein: 18g; Calories: 166; Fat: 8g; Carbohydrates: 5g; Fiber: 1g; Total sugar: 3g; Added sugar: 0g; Sodium: 252mg

QUICK CHICKEN BAKE

SERVES 4 // **PREP TIME**: 5 minutes // **COOK TIME**: 25 minutes

---

This moist and easy chicken bake can be assembled in about 15 minutes and thrown in the oven to finish cooking. I suggest serving it with a dash of fresh parsley and a teaspoon of Greek yogurt for extra flavor and creaminess. It is low in carbs and high in protein. Use ground turkey instead of chicken if you prefer. No extra salt is required, as canned tomatoes and cheese are salty.

---

1 teaspoon olive oil

½ teaspoon minced onion

1 garlic clove, minced

8 ounces ground chicken

1 cup frozen hash browns

½ cup canned diced tomatoes, with their juices

¼ cup shredded low-fat mozzarella cheese

1 tablespoon chopped fresh parsley (optional)

4 teaspoons nonfat plain Greek yogurt (optional)

1. Preheat the oven to 350°F.

2. In a small saucepan over medium heat, heat the oil. Add the onion and garlic. Sauté until golden, about 5 minutes.

3. Add the chicken, hash browns, and tomatoes with their juices and bring to a boil. Reduce the heat to maintain a simmer and cook, stirring occasionally, for 10 minutes, or until the liquid is fully reduced. Evenly divide the mixture among 4 (6-ounce) ramekins.

4. Top each with 1 tablespoon of mozzarella cheese.

5. Bake for 5 minutes, or until the cheese is melted and browned. Remove from the oven and top each with a sprinkle of parsley (if using) and 1 teaspoon of yogurt (if using) before serving. Enjoy.

COOKING TIP: Use a small baking dish instead of individual ramekins. Transfer all the ingredients to the dish, top with the cheese, and bake for 10 to 15 minutes. Let cool; then refrigerate, covered, for up to 3 days.

PER SERVING *(4 ounces)*: Protein: 13g; Calories: 159; Fat: 7g; Carbohydrates: 12g; Fiber: 1g; Total sugar: 1g; Added sugar: 0g; Sodium: 152mg

SOFT BASIL PESTO CHICKEN

SERVES 2 // **PREP TIME:** 5 minutes

5 Ingredients or Fewer
30 Minutes or Less
No Cook
One Pot

This recipe contains one of my favorite ingredients: basil pesto. Pesto is nutritious because it contains healthy fats from the olive oil and pine nuts. Although you can easily make your own basil pesto at home, I suggest buying your favorite premade pesto and keeping it in your refrigerator to add to dishes throughout the week. You can pair this recipe with soft crackers or make it into a wrap with romaine lettuce or butter lettuce leaves.

4 ounces low-sodium canned chicken, drained

1 tablespoon basil pesto

1. In a small bowl, mince the chicken with a fork.

2. Stir in the pesto and enjoy immediately.

STORAGE TIP: Make ahead and refrigerate this dish in an airtight container for up to 3 days.

PER SERVING *(2 ounces)*: Protein: 13g; Calories: 79; Fat: 2g; Carbohydrates: 1g; Fiber: 0g; Total sugar: <1g; Added sugar: 0g; Sodium: 154mg

GROUND CHICKEN AND CAULIFLOWER MASH

5 Ingredients or Fewer
30 Minutes or Less
One Pot

SERVES 2 // **PREP TIME:** 10 minutes // **COOK TIME:** 20 minutes

For this recipe, I suggest using a lean meat, like ground chicken or turkey. Adding water to the pan helps make the meat softer and juicier. I suggest choosing sweet bell peppers, such as red, yellow, or orange, to enhance the flavor. You can increase the portions of ingredients and enjoy this over several days. Be sure to prepare the Garlic Cauliflower and Potato Mash (page 172) ahead of time.

1 tablespoon olive oil

2 tablespoons diced red, yellow, or orange bell pepper

2 tablespoons diced white onion

¼ cup water

4 ounces ground chicken

½ cup Garlic Cauliflower and Potato Mash (page 172)

1. In a medium skillet over medium heat, heat the oil. Add the bell pepper and onion. Sauté for 5 to 10 minutes until the bell pepper is soft and the onion is golden brown.

2. Add the water and ground chicken. Mix well. Cook for 7 to 10 minutes, stirring frequently, until the meat is fully cooked with no pink remaining.

3. Spoon ½ cup of the chicken mixture over ¼ cup of cauliflower-potato mash and enjoy warm.

COOKING TIP: If you do not have Garlic Cauliflower and Potato Mash made, use store-bought mashed potatoes or canned vegetables such as potatoes or green beans.

PER SERVING *(2 ounces chicken and ½ cup cauliflower mash):* Protein: 12g; Calories: 229; Fat: 15g; Carbohydrates: 13g; Fiber: 2g; Total sugar: 2g; Added sugar: 0g; Sodium: 48mg

MEAT AND POTATO SALAD

SERVES 3 // **PREP TIME**: 10 minutes // **COOK TIME**: 30 minutes, plus time to cool and chill

Every family has its own version of homemade potato salad. I have seen variations in many cultures and cuisines. It is a complete meal that can be made with or without meat. You can use canned chicken in place of ham, or if you prefer plant-based ingredients, use canned peas or corn for protein and fiber.

1 small carrot

1 russet potato

1 hard-boiled egg, peeled and diced

½ cup diced cooked ham

2 tablespoons light mayonnaise

2 tablespoons diced scallion or fresh chives (optional)

Salt

Freshly ground black pepper

Garlic powder, for seasoning

1. In a medium saucepan, combine the carrot, potato, and enough cold water so the vegetables are covered by 2 to 3 inches. Bring to a boil over high heat and cook for about 30 minutes until soft. Let the vegetables cool; then peel and dice.

2. In a medium bowl, combine the diced potato and carrot, egg, ham, mayonnaise, and scallion (if using). Season with salt, pepper, and garlic powder to taste; then mix well to combine.

3. Chill before serving and enjoy cold.

STORAGE TIP: Refrigerate leftovers in an airtight container for up to 3 days.

PER SERVING (*4 ounces*): Protein: 9g; Calories: 136; Fat: 4g; Carbohydrates: 16g; Fiber: 1g; Total sugar: 2g; Added sugar: 0g; Sodium: 423mg

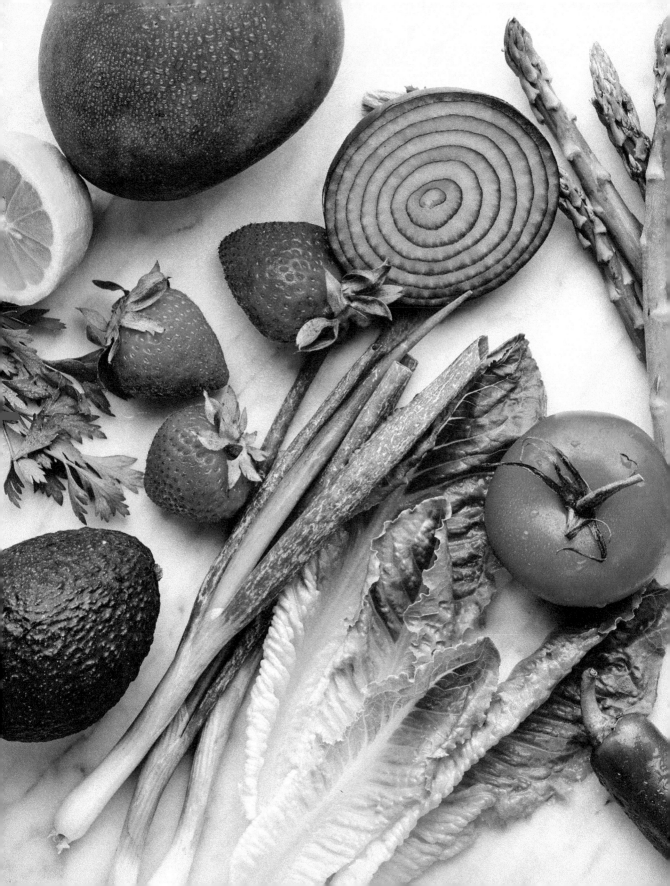

PART THREE

STAGE 4

RECIPES FOR LIFE

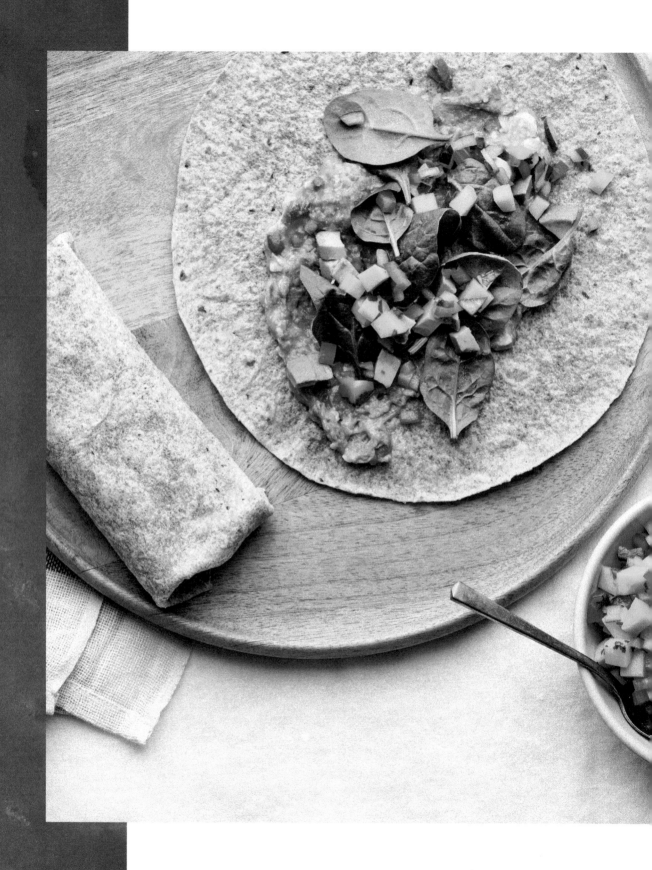

CHAPTER SIX

BREAKFAST

OATMEAL-PEAR SMOOTHIE

SERVES 1 // **PREP TIME:** 10 minutes

30 Minutes or Less
No Cook
One Pot

Hopefully you've already enjoyed the kefir smoothies from previous chapters. This recipe builds on that idea and includes ingredients that are high in fiber, such as rolled oats and fresh pear, as well as the calcium, protein, and probiotics kefir offers. It's an incredibly delicious fusion of simple flavors. Instead of sugar-free syrup, try honey.

8 ounces nonfat plain kefir

½ pear, diced

¼ cup rolled oats

1 tablespoon almond butter

1 teaspoon sugar-free syrup

½ teaspoon vanilla extract

¼ teaspoon ground cinnamon

1. In a blender, combine the kefir, pear, oats, almond butter, syrup, vanilla, and cinnamon.

2. Blend until smooth. Pour into a glass and enjoy.

STORAGE TIP: Refrigerate the remaining ½ pear for up to 1 day in an airtight container. Simply rub the cut side with lemon or pineapple juice to reduce browning.

PER SERVING *(1 smoothie; 10½ ounces):* Protein: 15g; Calories: 324; Fat: 12g; Carbohydrates: 41g; Fiber: 7g; Total sugar: 20g; Added sugar: 0g; Sodium: 94g

GREEK YOGURT, GRANOLA, AND BERRY PARFAIT

30 Minutes or Less
No Cook
One Pot

SERVES 1 // **PREP TIME**: 10 minutes

This fast, easy breakfast recipe can be assembled and enjoyed in the morning or taken to work for a protein-packed on-the-go parfait. It can also make a refreshing midday snack. The "granola" in this recipe is more of a deconstructed oat and nut mixture that can be endlessly changed up. I like to add sunflower seeds, which are high in vitamin E, antioxidants, and selenium.

½ cup nonfat plain Greek yogurt

1 tablespoon rolled oats

¼ cup fresh blueberries

¼ cup fresh raspberries

1 tablespoon chopped walnuts

1 tablespoon chopped pecans

1 teaspoon honey

1. Place the yogurt in a 6-ounce glass.

2. Top with the oats, blueberries, raspberries, walnuts, and pecans. Drizzle the honey on top. Enjoy immediately.

STORAGE TIP: You can prepare your own granola with rolled oats and your favorite nuts, as well as additional goodies such as coconut flakes, dried fruit, or fruit chips. Store it in an airtight container in a dry, dark place for up to 3 months. Use it in this parfait, a smoothie, or as a snack on its own.

PER SERVING *(8 ounces)*: Protein: 16g; Calories: 245; Fat: 11g; Carbohydrates: 25g; Fiber: 5g; Total sugar: 21g; Added sugar: 6g; Sodium: 46g

HIGH-PROTEIN PORRIDGE

SERVES 1 // **PREP TIME:** 5 minutes // **COOK TIME:** 25 minutes

5 Ingredients or Fewer
30 Minutes or Less
One Pot

There are many great variations on this traditional breakfast staple. In this recipe, I opt for walnuts, which are full of healthy fats, but use your favorite chopped, roasted nuts or seeds for crunch. You can also use any nut or seed butter you like as well as different jam flavors. Instead of raisins, mix it up with dried cranberries or cherries for tartness, but make sure no sugars have been added. The key is to add them while the porridge cooks so the fruit becomes soft and juicy. To save time, use quick cooking steel cut oats that can be ready in less than 10 minutes.

¾ cup water

¼ raw steel cut oats

1 tablespoon raisins, no sugar added

1 tablespoon chopped walnuts

1 tablespoon creamy almond butter

1 tablespoon sugar-free strawberry jam

1. In a small saucepan over high heat, bring the water to a boil.

2. Stir in the oats and raisins. Reduce the heat to low and simmer, uncovered, for 20 minutes, stirring regularly, until the oats have thickened and absorbed the water. Remove from the heat.

3. Stir in the walnuts. Let the mixture rest for 1 minute.

4. Top with the almond butter and strawberry jam. Enjoy warm.

POST-OP TIP: Oatmeal is very filling. I suggest waiting until you are at least six months post-op before adding it to your weekly breakfast rotation. Eat slowly, chew well, and stop when you feel full.

PER SERVING *(5½ ounces):* Protein: 10g; Calories: 338; Fat: 16g; Carbohydrates: 43g; Fiber: 7g; Total sugar: 7g; Added sugar: 0g; Sodium: 6g

EGG AND AVOCADO TOAST

SERVES 1 // **PREP TIME:** 5 minutes

5 Ingredients or Fewer
30 Minutes or Less
No Cook
One Pot

This quick breakfast toast is a helpful recipe to have in your back pocket for those mornings when time is short. At the start of the week, I like to hard-boil a few eggs and peel them for a quick grab-and-go snack or for use in recipes like this one. You can also purchase pre-boiled, peeled eggs. This toast is packed with protein from the egg and healthy fats from the avocado. The mustard adds a kick to the rich taste, and cilantro provides a pleasant fresh favor. To complete the meal, add your favorite fresh fruit.

1 slice whole-grain bread

1 teaspoon Dijon mustard

¼ avocado, peeled, pitted, and sliced

1 hard-boiled egg, cut into slices

1 tablespoon chopped fresh cilantro

Freshly ground black pepper (optional)

1. Toast the bread.

2. Spread the mustard over the toast; then top with the avocado slices.

3. Layer the egg slices on top. Sprinkle with cilantro, season with pepper (if using) to taste, and enjoy.

POST-OP TIP: Bread can be filling. I suggest waiting until you are at least six months post-op before adding it to your weekly breakfast rotation. Eat slowly, chew well, and stop when you feel full.

PER SERVING *(4 ounces)*: Protein: 12g; Calories: 239; Fat: 12g; Carbohydrates: 22g; Fiber: 6g; Total sugar: 3g; Added sugar: 0g; Sodium: 334g

OPEN-FACE FETA AND BASIL OMELET

30 Minutes or Less

SERVES 1 // **PREP TIME:** 10 minutes // **COOK TIME:** 5 minutes

I love to include vegetables in my breakfast because, when the day gets busy, they can be overlooked. This recipe calls for basil, but you can use spinach instead. I also like to make this open-face omelet with fresh dill or parsley or cherry tomatoes. There is no need for salt because feta is a salty cheese. To complete this breakfast, add fresh fruit or whole-grain toast.

1 large egg

2 tablespoons nonfat milk

1 tablespoon fresh basil leaves or ½ teaspoon dried basil

1 tablespoon chopped scallion

Freshly ground black pepper

1 teaspoon olive oil

½ ounce crumbled feta

1 small tomato, cut into wedges

1. In a small bowl, whisk the egg with a fork. Add the milk and beat lightly to combine.

2. Add the basil and scallion and season with pepper to taste. Mix well.

3. In a small pan over medium-low heat, heat the oil. Pour the egg mixture into the pan and sprinkle the feta and tomato on top. Cook for 3 to 4 minutes, or until the egg is set with no liquid remaining. Do not stir. Transfer to a plate and enjoy warm.

STORAGE TIP: Make extra omelets, cool them, and refrigerate in an airtight container for up to 3 days.

PER SERVING *(2½ ounces)*: Protein: 10g; Calories: 174; Fat: 13g; Carbohydrates: 6g; Fiber: 1g; Total sugar: 5g; Added sugar: 0g; Sodium: 234mg

BAKED EGG, PARM, AND SPINACH CUP

5 Ingredients or Fewer
30 Minutes or Less
One Pot

SERVES 1 // **PREP TIME**: 10 minutes // **COOK TIME**: 10 minutes

When you're in a hurry but want something quick and warm for breakfast, this dish delivers. Plus, it has vegetables—and what better way to start the day than with vegetables? Pair this egg cup with fresh fruit and whole-grain bread for a more filling meal. If you prefer runny eggs, bake for less time.

Nonstick cooking spray

¼ cup chopped fresh spinach

1 large egg

1 tablespoon nonfat milk

½ tomato, diced

1 tablespoon grated Parmesan cheese

Freshly ground black pepper

1. Preheat the oven to 400°F. Coat a 6-ounce ramekin with cooking spray.

2. Place the spinach in the ramekin; then crack the egg over the top.

3. Add the milk, tomato, and Parmesan cheese. Season with pepper to taste.

4. Bake for 10 minutes, or until set. Enjoy warm.

STORAGE TIP: Double or triple the recipe and make several egg cups at once. Let the egg cups cool; then tightly cover with plastic wrap and refrigerate for up 3 days. You can also cook several at once in a muffin tin (for 10 to 15 minutes until set), cool, and then refrigerate each in a sealed plastic zip-top bag for up to 3 days.

PER SERVING *(1 ramekin; 3 ounces)*: Protein: 9g; Calories: 112; Fat: 7g; Carbohydrates: 5g; Fiber: 1g; Total sugar: 3g; Added sugar: 0g; Sodium: 183g

LOX, EGG WHITE, AND AVOCADO SCRAMBLE

5 Ingredients or Fewer
30 Minutes or Less
One Pot

SERVES 1 // **PREP TIME:** 10 minutes // **COOK TIME:** 5 minutes

This is one of my favorite breakfast recipes, and I am excited for you to try it. Lox, a fillet of brined salmon, is high in omega-3 fatty acids, which many of us do not consume enough of. Egg whites are a complete protein, and avocado adds more healthy fats and creaminess to this luxurious dish. You can serve this on whole-grain toast, similar to a traditional bagel with lox.

1 teaspoon olive oil

2 large egg whites

Freshly ground
   black pepper

2 ounces lox

1½ teaspoons capers,
   drained and rinsed

1½ teaspoons chopped
   red onion

⅛ avocado, peeled, pitted,
   and cut into slices

1. In a small skillet over low heat, heat the oil. Add the egg whites and cook for 2 to 3 minutes, stirring occasionally, or until no liquid remains. Season with pepper to taste. Spoon the cooked eggs onto a plate.

2. Top with the lox, capers, red onion, and avocado. Enjoy immediately.

PER SERVING *(4 ounces)*: Protein: 17g; Calories: 167; Fat: 10g; Carbohydrates: 2g; Fiber: 1g; Total sugar: 1g; Added sugar: 0g; Sodium: 1334mg

RICOTTA AND SPINACH FRITTATA

5 Ingredients or Fewer
30 Minutes or Less

SERVES 1 // **PREP TIME**: 10 minutes // **COOK TIME**: 15 minutes

This ricotta-filled frittata is an easy breakfast or brunch that can be ready in about 25 minutes and bursts with flavor from fresh vegetables. I always encourage patients to add vegetables to any dishes they can. You can also use frozen spinach if you have some on hand. To make this meal more filling, pair it with fresh fruit or whole-grain toast.

1½ teaspoons olive oil

1 tablespoon diced onion

1 tablespoon diced mushroom

¼ cup fresh spinach

1 large egg

2 tablespoons part-skim ricotta

Salt

Freshly ground black pepper

1. In a small skillet over medium-low heat, heat the oil. Add the onion and sauté for 5 to 7 minutes until golden brown.

2. Add the mushroom and spinach to the skillet. Cook for about 5 minutes until the mushroom is soft and the spinach wilts.

3. In a small bowl, whisk the egg with a fork until smooth.

4. Add the ricotta to the skillet and pour the egg over the top. Season with salt and pepper to taste. Cook for 3 to 4 minutes, without stirring, or until the egg is firm. Serve warm and enjoy.

STORAGE TIP: Let the frittata cool completely; then refrigerate in an airtight container for up to 3 days.

PER SERVING *(4½ ounces)*: Protein: 10g; Calories: 177; Fat: 14g; Carbohydrates: 3g; Fiber: <1g; Total sugar: 1g; Added sugar: 0g; Sodium: 92mg

HEARTY WHOLE-GRAIN BREAKFAST BURRITO

30 Minutes or Less
One Pot

SERVES 1 // **PREP TIME:** 10 minutes // **COOK TIME:** 10 minutes

I couldn't write a cookbook and not include a breakfast burrito recipe. With just a few simple, wholesome, healthy ingredients, this complete, nutritionally balanced meal takes no time to make and is full of fiber from the beans, whole-grain tortilla, and vegetables. Enjoy this burrito with your favorite salsa.

½ teaspoon olive oil or olive oil spray

1 large egg

¼ cup fat-free refried beans

1 tablespoon shredded low-fat Cheddar cheese

1 medium (8-inch) whole-grain tortilla

⅛ avocado, peeled, pitted, and diced

¼ cup fresh spinach

Salsa, for serving (optional)

1. In a small skillet over medium-low heat, heat the oil.

2. Crack the egg into the skillet and cook, scrambling it with a spatula, for 1 to 2 minutes, or until the egg is almost cooked.

3. Add the beans and cook for 2 to 3 minutes to warm.

4. Add the Cheddar cheese, mix well, and cook for 1 to 2 minutes more until the cheese melts.

5. Warm the tortilla on a plate in the microwave on high power for about 1 minute.

6. Spoon the eggs, beans, and cheese onto the warm tortilla. Top with avocado, spinach, and salsa (if using). Fold into a burrito and enjoy.

STORAGE TIP: Double or triple the burrito filling and, once cool, refrigerate in an airtight container for up to 3 days. When ready to eat, warm a tortilla as you reheat the filling; then spoon the filling into the tortilla and top with spinach, avocado, and salsa.

PER SERVING *(5½ ounces)*: Protein: 14g; Calories: 256; Fat: 12g; Carbohydrates: 23g; Fiber: 14g; Total sugar: 1g; Added sugar: 0g; Sodium: 525mg

TURKEY, CHEESE, AND HASH BROWN MINI-BAKE

30 Minutes or Less
One Pot

SERVES 2 // **PREP TIME:** 10 minutes // **COOK TIME:** 20 minutes

This recipe is moderate in calories, high in protein, and delicious served hot. You can swap turkey for ground chicken or the meat of your choice. To make this recipe even faster, use premade meat patties, burgers, meatloaf, or sausages. Or try other ground meat recipes from this book, which can be made ahead and used in this breakfast bake—just reduce the baking time by half. Look for hash browns in the frozen vegetable aisle of your grocery store. For less heat, use sliced olives instead of green chiles.

Olive oil spray

4 ounces lean ground turkey

Salt

Freshly ground black pepper

Onion powder, for seasoning

Garlic powder, for seasoning

1 tablespoon canned diced green chiles

½ cup frozen hash browns

2 tablespoons shredded low-fat Cheddar cheese

1. Preheat the oven 425°F.

2. Coat 2 (6-ounce) ramekins with olive oil spray.

3. Evenly divide the ground turkey between the prepared ramekins. Season with salt, pepper, onion powder, and garlic powder to taste. Top each with 1½ teaspoons of green chiles and ¼ cup of hash browns.

4. Bake for 10 to 15 minutes, or until the turkey is fully cooked with no pink remaining.

5. Top each with 1 tablespoon of Cheddar cheese and bake for 3 to 5 minutes more until the cheese melts. Enjoy warm.

COOKING TIP: Double or triple this recipe and cook it in a casserole dish or muffin tin for extra portions you can reheat and eat throughout the week.

PER SERVING *(1 ramekin; 4 ounces)*: Protein: 18g; Calories: 179; Fat: 7g; Carbohydrates: 10g; Fiber: 1g; Total sugar: <1g; Added sugar: 0g; Sodium: 154g

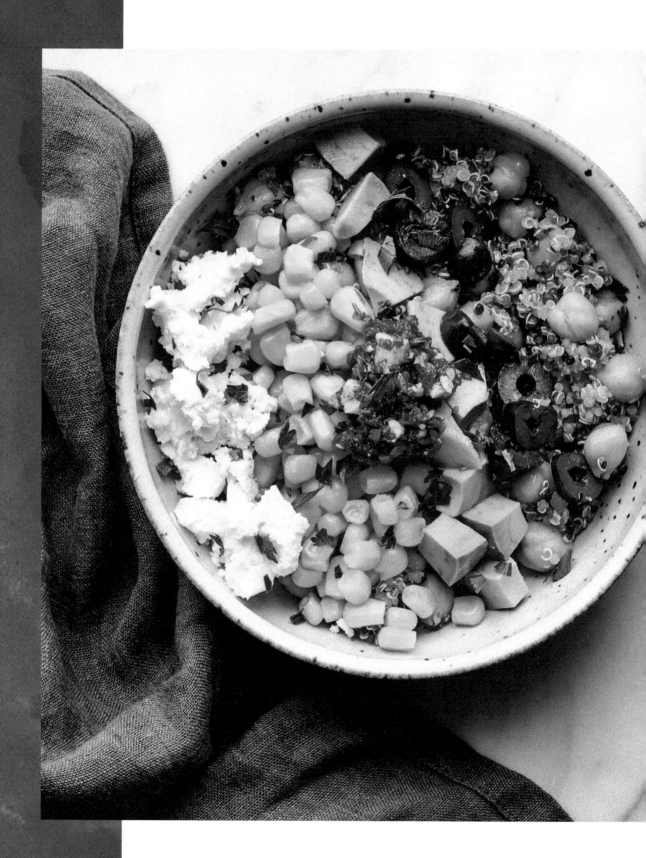

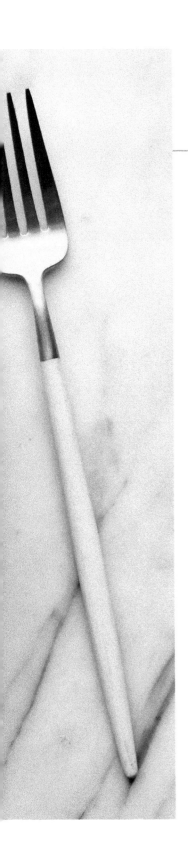

CHAPTER SEVEN

VEGETARIAN

DAIRY-FREE DATE AND BANANA SHAKE

SERVES 1 // **PREP TIME:** 10 minutes

5 Ingredients or Fewer
30 Minutes or Less
No Cook
One Pot

This simple shake is a great way to get your fruits in without adding sugar or sweetener—because dates are naturally sweet. This is also a great option for those who choose not to consume dairy. Typically, almond milk has no protein, so I suggest using either high-protein almond milk (I like Orgain brand) or adding unflavored protein powder. But if you prefer dairy, use kefir or buttermilk instead. Unlike shakes from the liquid diet stage, you can add more fruits and oats now.

1 small banana, fresh or frozen

¼ cup rolled oats

1½ tablespoons almond butter

1 pitted date

1 cup unsweetened vanilla almond milk

Unflavored protein powder (10 grams; optional)

3 or 4 ice cubes

1. In a blender, combine the banana, oats, almond butter, date, milk, protein powder (if using), and ice.

2. Blend until smooth. Enjoy immediately.

COOKING TIP: Before using, soak the date in hot water for 5 minutes to make sure it is soft and juicy.

PER SERVING *(12½ ounces)*: Protein: 10g; Calories: 361; Fat: 17g; Carbohydrates: 48g; Fiber: 8g; Total sugar: 18g; Added sugar: 0g; Sodium: 174mg

GREEN KEFIR SMOOTHIE

SERVES 1 // **PREP TIME:** 10 minutes

Unlike smoothies in the liquid stage, you can now add fresh fruits and vegetables to increase fiber intake. Some people find it difficult to eat fruits and vegetables during the day, so smoothies are a great way to fill the gap. This is a complete meal full of nutrients: The kefir offers calcium, protein, and probiotics; the apple and date lend natural sweetness and fiber; the veggies provide antioxidants and fiber; and the avocado gives this smoothie healthy and filling fats. Remember to soak the date for extra softness before using.

1 cup nonfat plain kefir

1 pitted date

½ apple, cored and chopped

¼ cup fresh spinach

½ small cucumber, chopped

⅛ avocado, peeled and pitted

1. In a blender, combine the kefir, date, apple, spinach, cucumber, and avocado.

2. Blend until smooth. Enjoy immediately.

PER SERVING *(12½ ounces)*: Protein: 10g; Calories: 203; Fat: 5g; Carbohydrates: 33g; Fiber: 5g; Total sugar: 26g; Added sugar: 0g; Sodium: 101mg

CHICKPEA SALAD

SERVES 1 // **PREP TIME:** 15 minutes

Chickpeas, also called garbanzo beans, are a great source of protein and fiber for those looking to add more plant-based protein into their diet. They are shelf stable and great to have on hand for adding to salads, soups, and more. There's no need for dressing on this salad; the avocado provides creaminess.

½ cup canned low-sodium chickpeas, drained and rinsed

⅓ avocado, peeled, pitted, and diced

1 tomato, diced

1 Persian cucumber, diced

1 tablespoon chopped fresh cilantro

1 tablespoon chopped scallion (optional)

½ ounce feta cheese

1. In a medium bowl, combine the chickpeas, avocado, tomato, cucumber, cilantro, and scallion (if using).

2. Crumble the feta cheese into the bowl. Mix well and enjoy.

POST-OP TIP: This recipe has a lot of fiber. Drinking extra water 30 to 45 minutes after eating this salad will help digestion. This meal is great if you're struggling with post-op constipation.

STORAGE TIP: To make ahead, refrigerate the diced cucumber and tomato in separate containers for up to 2 days. Leftover canned chickpeas can be refrigerated in an airtight container for up to 3 days. When ready to eat, mix all the ingredients and add fresh or frozen avocado.

PER SERVING *(5½ ounces)*: Protein: 10g; Calories: 253; Fat: 13g; Carbohydrates: 32g; Fiber: 12g; Total sugar: 7g; Added sugar: 0g; Sodium: 177mg

EASY CAPRESE SALAD

SERVES 1 // **PREP TIME:** 10 minutes

5 Ingredients or Fewer
30 Minutes or Less
No Cook
One Pot

Here is an easy twist on the classic caprese salad. Fresh basil is not always available, so use basil pesto instead or even olive oil. I suggest trying flavored olive oils like basil or oregano. Pair this salad with crackers or white beans to make a complete meal.

2 ounces fresh mozzarella cheese, cut into ¼-inch-thick rounds

½ large tomato, cut into ¼-inch-thick rounds

1 teaspoon basil pesto

1 teaspoon aged balsamic vinegar

Salt

Freshly ground black pepper

1. Arrange the mozzarella slices on a plate.

2. Arrange the tomato slices over the mozzarella slices.

3. Dot the salad with pesto, and then drizzle with vinegar. Season with salt and pepper to taste and enjoy immediately.

COOKING TIP: If you have fresh basil leaves on hand, add a few to this salad, on top of the tomato slices. Omit the pesto and drizzle with a little olive oil and balsamic vinegar.

PER SERVING *(2½ ounces)*: Protein: 11g; Calories: 204; Fat: 15g; Carbohydrates: 5g; Fiber: 1g; Total sugar: 3g; Added sugar: 0g; Sodium: 219mg

STUFFED PORTABELLA MUSHROOM

SERVES 1 // **PREP TIME:** 10 minutes // **COOK TIME:** 20 minutes

You can do so many things with portabella mushrooms, a versatile ingredient in the vegetarian diet. Pair this dish with Garlic Cauliflower and Potato Mash (page 172) or a side of white beans for added protein and fiber. You can also swap basil for oregano or paprika if you prefer. Follow the directions carefully to learn how to cook mushrooms correctly.

1 medium or large porta-bella mushroom

1 teaspoon olive oil

1 large egg

1 ounce shredded low-fat mozzarella cheese

1 tablespoon chopped artichoke heart

1 tablespoon shredded Parmesan cheese

Chopped fresh basil leaves, for garnish (optional)

1. Preheat the oven to 375°F.

2. Trim off the mushroom stem; then scrape out the gills with a spoon and discard. Brush the oil all over the mushroom and place it on a baking sheet, stem-side up. Bake for 5 minutes.

3. While the mushroom bakes, in a small bowl, stir together the egg, mozzarella cheese, and artichoke heart until well combined.

4. Remove the baking sheet from the oven; check for any water that may have pooled inside the mushroom and drain. (Mushrooms are naturally watery.)

5. Spoon the egg and cheese mixture into the mushroom. Sprinkle with the Parmesan cheese. Bake for 10 to 15 minutes more, or until the egg is set and the cheese is melted. Remove from the oven, sprinkle with basil (if using), and enjoy.

COOKING TIP: You can also stuff the mushrooms with vegetarian meat alternatives mixed with the cheese.

PER SERVING *(4 ounces)*: Protein: 17g; Calories: 248; Fat: 17g; Carbohydrates: 9g; Fiber: 3g; Total sugar: 4g; Added sugar: 0g; Sodium: 354mg

RICOTTA-STUFFED JALAPEÑO PEPPERS

5 Ingredients or Fewer
30 Minutes or Less

SERVES 1 // **PREP TIME**: 10 minutes // **COOK TIME**: 20 minutes

This recipe is easy to prepare ahead, freeze, and then throw into the oven when you're hungry. It is a soft, cheesy treat for anyone who likes spicy foods. Sprinkle bacon crumbs on top for extra flavor. For a complete meal, pair the stuffed peppers with white beans or Garlic Cauliflower and Potato Mash (page 172).

1 tablespoon chopped scallion

1 tablespoon chopped fresh cilantro

2 tablespoons part-skim ricotta

Salt

Ground cumin, for seasoning (optional)

2 jalapeño peppers, halved lengthwise and seeded

1 ounce low-fat Monterey Jack cheese, cut into 4 slices

1. Preheat the oven to 375°F. Line a baking sheet with aluminum foil. Set aside.

2. In a small bowl, stir together the scallion, cilantro, and ricotta. Season with salt and cumin (if using) to taste and stir again. Spoon the filling into the jalapeño halves and place 1 slice of Jack cheese on top of each filled half. Place the stuffed peppers on the prepared baking sheet.

3. Bake for 15 to 20 minutes (15 for crispier peppers; 20 minutes for softer peppers). Remove from the oven and let the peppers cool for a few minutes before enjoying.

COOKING TIP: Double or triple this recipe and refrigerate the stuffed peppers in an airtight container for up to 3 days or freeze in a freezer-safe plastic zip-top bag, tightly sealed with as much air as possible pressed out, for up to 2 months. Thaw before cooking.

PER SERVING *(3 ounces)*: Protein: 11g; Calories: 158; Fat: 11g; Carbohydrates: 4g; Fiber: 1g; Total sugar: 2g; Added sugar: 0g; Sodium: 203mg

PLANT-BASED PROTEIN BOWL

30 Minutes or Less
No Cook
One Pot

SERVES 1 // **PREP TIME**: 15 minutes

This bowl is one of my favorite lunches because it's full of plant-based ingredients and fiber. You can make several variations: Instead of quinoa, try wild rice, farro, or buckwheat. You can also use different beans, like black beans or white beans, and if you don't like olives, substitute artichoke hearts. If you don't have basil pesto, try Sundried Tomato Pesto (page 169). For added protein, top the bowl with an egg (boiled, fried, or poached).

¼ cooked quinoa (store-bought or homemade; see Herb Quinoa, page 171)

¼ cup canned low-sodium chickpeas, drained and rinsed

1 teaspoon basil pesto

¼ cup canned corn, drained and rinsed

½ ounce feta cheese, crumbled

3 Kalamata olives, pitted and sliced

⅛ avocado, peeled, pitted, and cut into slices

Chopped fresh parsley, for garnish (optional)

1. In a small bowl, stir together the quinoa, chickpeas, and pesto. Mix well.

2. Top with the corn, feta, and olives.

3. Garnish with avocado and parsley (if using) and enjoy.

STORAGE TIP: Prepare the ingredients ahead so all you have to do is assemble and eat. Cook a large batch of quinoa and refrigerate it for up to 3 days to use across recipes, or buy precooked quinoa at many grocery stores. When you open canned vegetables and feta, refrigerate whatever you don't use in airtight containers for up to 3 days.

PER SERVING *(6½ ounces)*: Protein: 9g; Calories: 267; Fat: 14g; Carbohydrates: 29g; Fiber: 6g; Total sugar: 5g; Added sugar: 0g; Sodium: 534mg

VEGETARIAN TACO WITH MANGO SALSA

30 Minutes or Less
One Pot

SERVES 1 // **PREP TIME:** 10 minutes // **COOK TIME:** 10 minutes

This taco is easy to make and both juicy and rich in flavor. If you prefer not to use a tortilla, wrap your taco in a romaine lettuce or butter lettuce leaf. Instead of black beans, try chickpeas or a vegan meat substitute. When buying canned vegetables or beans, opt for low-sodium versions. If you can't find low-sodium choices at your grocer, rinse the veggies or beans under cold water to reduce their sodium content before using.

1 teaspoon olive oil

¼ cup canned black beans, drained and rinsed

¼ cup canned corn, drained and rinsed

1 small (6-inch) whole-grain tortilla

1 tablespoon Mango Salsa (page 168)

1 tablespoon shredded lettuce

1 tablespoon nonfat plain Greek yogurt

⅛ avocado, peeled, pitted, and cut into slices (optional)

1 tablespoon shredded low-fat cheese of choice (optional)

1. In a medium skillet over low heat, heat the oil. Add the black beans and corn and cook for 5 minutes until warmed.

2. While the beans and corn cook, warm the tortilla on a plate in the microwave on high power for about 1 minute.

3. Spoon the corn and bean mixture into the warmed tortilla and top with mango salsa, lettuce, yogurt, and avocado (if using). Sprinkle with cheese (if using) and enjoy.

COOKING TIP: If you don't have Mango Salsa ready, use your favorite salsa.

PER SERVING *(6½ ounces)*: Protein: 9g; Calories: 232; Fat: 7g; Carbohydrates: 34g; Fiber: 16g; Total sugar: 6g; Added sugar: 0g; Sodium: 290mg

QUICK CHEESE AND VEGGIE QUESADILLA

5 Ingredients or Fewer
30 Minutes or Less
One Pot

SERVES 1 // **PREP TIME:** 5 minutes // **COOK TIME:** 5 minutes

Who doesn't like a good cheese quesadilla for lunch or dinner? I suggest adding spinach—get those veggies in any way you can. The Mango Salsa (page 168) offers even more veggies and fruit. You can also use a corn tortilla, if you prefer, instead of whole grain. Pair this dish with a small salad for a filling and even more veggie-packed meal.

1 medium (8-inch) whole-grain tortilla

1½ ounces shredded pepper Jack cheese

¼ cup fresh spinach

¼ cup Mango Salsa (page 168)

1. In a small skillet over low heat, warm the tortilla for about 1 minute.

2. Top with the pepper Jack cheese and spinach. Cook for 3 to 4 minutes until the cheese melts. Fold the tortilla in half.

3. Serve warm topped with mango salsa, and enjoy.

PER SERVING *(5 ounces)*: Protein: 13g; Calories: 293; Fat: 15g; Carbohydrates: 29g; Fiber: 12g; Total sugar: 13g; Added sugar: 0g; Sodium: 481mg

CRUNCHY HUMMUS AND PESTO WRAP

30 Minutes or Less
No Cook
One Pot

SERVES 1 // **PREP TIME**: 10 minutes

When I'm looking for something simple to whip up for lunch, dinner, or even a filling snack, this wrap is my go-to choice. The hummus and pesto make it easy to eat, and the veggies provide crunch, texture, vitamins, and minerals. It is very filling, but if you think you need more, serve the wrap with fruit or a side of yogurt.

1 medium (8-inch) whole-grain tortilla

2 tablespoons hummus

1½ teaspoons Sundried Tomato Pesto (page 169)

5 thin slices red bell pepper

½ cup shredded lettuce

1 slice pepper Jack cheese

1. Place the tortilla on a plate. Spread the hummus and pesto over the tortilla.

2. Add a layer of bell pepper and sprinkle with lettuce and cheese. Fold the tortilla into a wrap and enjoy.

COOKING TIP: Try this with basil pesto if you don't have Sundried Tomato Pesto made. Also, try different vegetables, such as tomato, cucumber, or radish for variety.

PER SERVING *(5 ounces)*: Protein: 11g; Calories: 345; Fat: 19g; Carbohydrates: 32g; Fiber: 6g; Total sugar: 2g; Added sugar: 0g; Sodium: 593mg

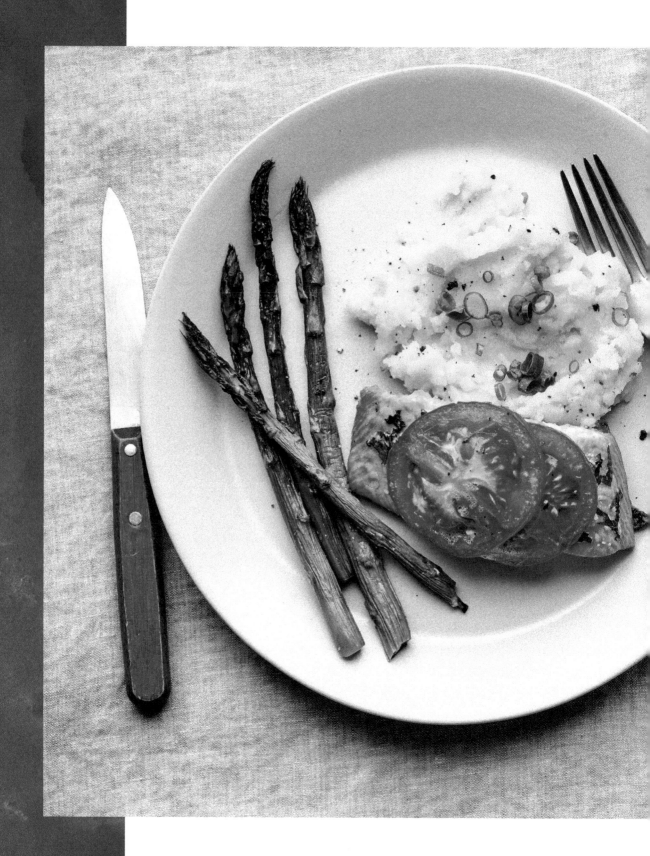

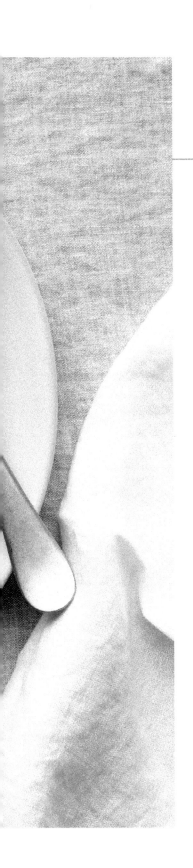

CHAPTER EIGHT

SEAFOOD

"MAYO-LESS" MEDITERRANEAN TUNA SALAD

SERVES 2 // **PREP TIME**: 10 minutes

This gourmet tuna salad is full of healthy fats and omega-3s from the tuna and is a breeze to put together. I recommend enjoying it with whole-grain crackers for a quick and healthy snack or on whole-grain toast or over a bed of lettuce for a satisfying lunch or dinner. Try it with a Parmesan Crisp (page 170), too.

4 ounces canned oil-packed tuna, drained

2 tablespoons capers, drained and rinsed

1 tablespoon finely chopped red onion

1 tablespoon finely chopped fresh dill, or 1 teaspoon dried dill

2 tablespoons Dijon mustard

» In a medium bowl, stir together the tuna, capers, red onion, dill, and Dijon until well combined and enjoy.

COOKING TIP: If you don't have capers, use chopped olives. For a low-sodium option, consider no-salt-added tuna.

STORAGE TIP: This salad can be made ahead and refrigerated in an airtight container for up to 3 days.

PER SERVING *(2½ ounces)*: Protein: 17g; Calories: 132; Fat: 6g; Carbohydrates: 2g; Fiber: 1g; Total sugar: <1g; Added sugar: 0g; Sodium: 798mg

TUNA WRAP

SERVES 1 // **PREP TIME:** 10 minutes

For this wrap I suggest using a corn or whole-grain tortilla instead of flour for added fiber. Avocado makes this wrap creamy, and vegetables add freshness and crunch. You can also swap canned tuna for canned salmon. I suggest selecting a canned fish with no added salt.

1 medium (8-inch) whole-grain tortilla

¼ avocado, peeled, pitted, and mashed

2 ounces canned oil-packed tuna, drained

5 cucumber slices

¼ red bell pepper, cut into slices

1 tablespoon chopped fresh cilantro

1. Place the tortilla on a plate and spread the mashed avocado over it.

2. Layer on the tuna, cucumber, red bell pepper, and cilantro. Wrap and enjoy.

PER SERVING *(5 ounces)*: Protein: 22g; Calories: 320; Fat: 13g; Carbohydrates: 31g; Fiber: 7g; Total sugar: 3g; Added sugar: 0g; Sodium: 545mg

SHRIMP POKE BOWL

30 Minutes or Less
One Pot

SERVES 1 // **PREP TIME**: 10 minutes // **COOK TIME**: 10 minutes

You can make a poke bowl with any seafood: crab, fish, scallop, or shrimp. The vegetables, soy, and fruit add antioxidants, vitamins, and minerals, keeping the calories low but delivering a lot of flavor. Most grocery stores sell pre-cooked edamame (soybeans and a source of plant-based protein) fresh or frozen as well as nori (dried seaweed) in shredded or sheet form. If you don't have sesame oil, use more olive oil.

1 teaspoon olive oil

2 ounces fresh shrimp, peeled and deveined

¼ cup cooked brown rice

1 tablespoon cooked edamame

1 teaspoon soy sauce

1 teaspoon sesame oil

2 tablespoons Mango Salsa (page 168)

1 teaspoon chopped scallion

½ teaspoon sesame seeds (optional)

Chopped fresh cilantro, for garnish (optional)

Shredded nori, for garnish (optional)

1. In a small pan over medium heat, heat the oil. Add the shrimp and cook for 7 to 10 minutes, flipping to ensure that each piece is cooked on all sides. Transfer to a small bowl.

2. Add the brown rice and edamame to the shrimp. Drizzle with soy sauce and sesame oil. Mix to combine.

3. Top with the mango salsa, scallion, sesame seeds (if using), cilantro (if using), and nori (if using). Enjoy immediately.

STORAGE TIP: Double the recipe and let the leftover shrimp cool. Refrigerate each ingredient in a separate container for up to 3 days When ready to eat, mix everything together in a bowl.

PER SERVING *(4 ounces)*: Protein: 13g; Calories: 226; Fat: 11g; Carbohydrates: 22g; Fiber: 2g; Total sugar: 7g; Added sugar: 0g; Sodium: 445mg

GARLIC-OLIVE OIL SHRIMP WITH QUINOA

5 Ingredients or Fewer
30 Minutes or Less
One Pot

SERVES 2 // **PREP TIME:** 10 minutes // **COOK TIME:** 15 minutes

This recipe requires only a handful of ingredients and cooks in just 15 minutes—perfect for a busy evening. Plus, there's no need for greasy butter sauce; olive oil is just as delicious and healthier. Try herb-infused olive oils for added flavor. This recipe uses Herb Quinoa (page 171). If you don't have quinoa handy, serve the shrimp in lettuce wraps or over a bed of lettuce instead. You can also add this shrimp to your salads and tacos.

2 teaspoons olive oil

2 garlic cloves, minced

4 ounces fresh shrimp, peeled and deveined

½ cup Herb Quinoa (page 171)

1 tomato, cut into slices

1 lemon, cut into wedges (optional)

1. In a small pan over medium heat, heat the oil. Add the garlic and sauté for 5 minutes until brown.

2. Add the shrimp and cook for 7 to 10 minutes, flipping to ensure that each piece is cooked on all sides. Remove the shrimp from the pan and divide between 2 plates, reserving the pan drippings.

3. Add ¼ cup of quinoa to each plate and drizzle with garlic oil from the pan.

4. Top with the tomato slices, serve with a lemon wedge (if using) for squeezing, and enjoy.

STORAGE TIP: Double or triple the shrimp in this recipe and refrigerate it in an airtight container for up to 3 days.

PER SERVING *(4 ounces)*: Protein: 10g; Calories: 135; Fat: 7g; Carbohydrates: 10g; Fiber: 1g; Total sugar: 2g; Added sugar: 0g; Sodium: 425mg

PESTO-PARMESAN SHRIMP AND BROCCOLI

30 Minutes or Less
One Pot

SERVES 2 // **PREP TIME:** 10 minutes // **COOK TIME:** 15 minutes

Pesto pairs well with just about anything—especially shrimp. If you want to add a healthy carb, I suggest serving the shrimp with brown or wild rice. To save time, purchase precooked brown rice in the frozen section of the grocery store, or pair this dish with another grain, such as Herb Quinoa (page 171).

1 tablespoon basil pesto

1 teaspoon minced garlic

4 ounces fresh shrimp, peeled and deveined

½ cup diced broccoli

½ cup cooked brown rice

1 tablespoon shredded Parmesan cheese

1. In a medium pan over medium heat, combine the pesto, garlic, and shrimp. Cook for 5 minutes, turning the shrimp until it is cooked on all sides.

2. Add the broccoli and cover the pan. Cook for 5 to 10 minutes more, depending on how soft you like your broccoli.

3. Divide the shrimp and broccoli mixture between 2 plates and add ¼ cup of brown rice on the side. Sprinkle with the Parmesan cheese and enjoy.

COOKING TIP: If you don't have pesto, cook the shrimp in basil-flavored olive oil with fresh garlic to taste.

STORAGE TIP: Refrigerate extra portions in an airtight container for up to 3 days.

PER SERVING *(5½ ounces)*: Protein: 11g; Calories: 154; Fat: 6g; Carbohydrates: 16g; Fiber: 2g; Total sugar: 1g; Added sugar: 0g; Sodium: 548mg

SCALLOPS WITH WHITE BEANS AND SUNDRIED TOMATO PESTO

5 Ingredients or Fewer
30 Minutes or Less
One Pot

SERVES 1 // **PREP TIME:** 5 minutes // **COOK TIME:** 10 minutes

I had to include a scallop recipe in this book. Tender and juicy, scallops are a great source of lean protein. They are also easy to make, and you can find them fresh or frozen in most grocery stores. If you use frozen scallops, thaw them completely before cooking. If you do not have Sundried Tomato Pesto (page 169) on hand, use olive oil with garlic or basil pesto instead.

1 teaspoon olive oil

2 ounces raw scallops

2 tablespoons Sundried Tomato Pesto (page 169)

½ cup fresh spinach

¼ cup canned white beans, drained and rinsed

1. In a small pan over medium heat, heat the oil. Add the scallops and cook for 2 minutes. Flip and cook for 2 minutes more.

2. Add the pesto to the pan and cook for 2 minutes, or until the scallops are golden brown on each side.

3. Place the spinach and white beans on a plate and top with the cooked scallops and pesto. Enjoy.

COOKING TIP: Scallops cook quickly. Do not overcook them or they will be rubbery.

PER SERVING *(5 ounces)*: Protein: 13g; Calories: 367; Fat: 28g; Carbohydrates: 18g; Fiber: 5g; Total sugar: 3g; Added sugar: 0g; Sodium: 427mg

BAKED CHEESY HALIBUT WITH AVOCADO

*5 Ingredients or Fewer
30 Minutes or Less
One Pot*

SERVES 1 // **PREP TIME**: 10 minutes // **COOK TIME**: 20 minutes

I had a dish similar to this in a fancy restaurant, and I realized how easy it is to make. I love to make it with pepper Jack cheese, but you can use any white cheese you like, and if you prefer cod, use that instead of halibut. This recipe calls for a side of wild rice, which you can make in advance and refrigerate to serve alongside lunch or dinner (or buy frozen and heat it quickly in the microwave). However, this dish also pairs perfectly with Garlic Cauliflower and Potato Mash (page 172).

2 ounces halibut

1 tablespoon shredded pepper Jack cheese, or ½ slice

⅛ avocado, peeled, pitted, and thinly sliced

5 cucumber slices

¼ cup cooked wild rice

1. Preheat the oven to 400°F. Line a baking sheet with nonstick aluminum foil.

2. Place the fish on the right side of the prepared baking sheet. Fold the left side of the foil over the fish, pinching the edges to create a packet.

3. Bake for 10 to 13 minutes, or until the fish flakes easily with a fork. Remove the fish from the oven, unwrap it, and top with the Jack cheese. Bake, uncovered, for 3 minutes, or until the cheese melts.

4. Transfer the fish to a plate and top with the avocado. Arrange the cucumber slices and wild rice on the side. Enjoy.

COOKING TIP: For a lower-carb option, omit the wild rice and place the fish on a lettuce leaf.

PER SERVING (*5 ounces*): Protein: 15g; Calories: 167; Fat: 7g; Carbohydrates: 13g; Fiber: 2g; Total sugar: 1g; Added sugar: 0g; Sodium: 112mg

COD WITH MANGO SALSA

SERVES 1 // **PREP TIME**: 10 minutes // **COOK TIME**: 15 minutes

5 Ingredients or Fewer
30 Minutes or Less
One Pot

Although this recipe calls for cod, I have made it with a variety of white fish, including halibut, ono, and tilapia. It tastes refreshing and juicy with all. If you don't have time to make Mango Salsa (page 168) or don't have any prepped, use your favorite tomato salsa. To save time, look for precooked rice in the frozen section of most grocery stores—just microwave it for a few minutes before serving.

2 ounces cod

1 teaspoon olive oil

Salt

Freshly ground
    black pepper

2 tablespoons Mango
    Salsa (page 168)

¼ cup cooked brown rice

1. Preheat the oven to 400°F. Line a baking sheet with nonstick aluminum foil.

2. Place the fish on the right side of the prepared baking sheet. Drizzle the fish with oil and season with salt and pepper to taste. Fold the left side of the foil over the fish, pinching the edges together to create a packet.

3. Bake for 15 minutes, or until the fish flakes easily with a fork. Transfer the fish to a plate and top with mango salsa. Serve with brown rice and enjoy.

PER SERVING *(5 ounces)*: Protein: 12g; Calories: 175; Fat: 6g; Carbohydrates: 20g; Fiber: 2g; Total sugar: 6g; Added sugar: 0g; Sodium: 55mg

BAKED SALMON AND ASPARAGUS WITH BASIL AND TOMATO

5 Ingredients or Fewer
30 Minutes or Less
One Pot

SERVES 2 // **PREP TIME:** 10 minutes // **COOK TIME:** 20 minutes

Salmon is full of healthy fats and is a naturally soft fish. By adding acidic tomato, the salmon will be even softer and easier to eat. Paired with asparagus drizzled with olive oil and garlic, this fish dish will easily become one of your go-to favorites. Serve it with your favorite starch, such as ¼ cup of cooked brown rice or Garlic Cauliflower and Potato Mash (page 172), for a more filling meal.

2 (2-ounce) salmon fillets

1 tomato, cut into 4 slices

4 fresh basil leaves, chopped, or ¼ teaspoon dried basil

Salt

8 asparagus spears, woody ends removed

1 teaspoon olive oil

¼ teaspoon dried garlic, or 1 garlic clove, smashed

2 lemon wedges (optional)

1. Preheat the oven to 400°F. Line a baking sheet with nonstick aluminum foil.

2. Place the salmon on the right side of the prepared baking sheet. Top each fillet with 2 tomato slices and then the chopped basil. Season with salt to taste.

3. Place the asparagus next to the fish and drizzle it with the oil. Season with the garlic and salt to taste.

4. Fold the left side of the foil over the salmon and asparagus and pinch the edges together to create a packet.

5. Bake for 15 to 20 minutes, or until the salmon flakes easily with a fork. Transfer the salmon and veggies to a plate. Pour the juices left in the foil over the fish and asparagus, and serve with a lemon wedge (if using). Enjoy warm.

COOKING TIP: Top the salmon and asparagus with basil pesto.

PER SERVING *(3 ounces)*: Protein: 13g; Calories: 89; Fat: 3g; Carbohydrates: 5g; Fiber: 2g; Total sugar: 4g; Added sugar: 0g; Sodium: 89mg

YOGURT-DILL SALMON AND BAKED POTATO

30 Minutes or Less

SERVES 2 // **PREP TIME:** 5 minutes // **COOK TIME:** 20 minutes

The combination of Greek yogurt and dill mimics fresh tzatziki sauce and provides additional protein for this meal. It also makes the salmon very creamy and flavorful. Put the potatoes in the oven first as they may take longer to cook.

1 small russet potato, cut into thin wedges or slices (about ½ cup)

1 teaspoon olive oil

Garlic powder, for seasoning

Salt

Freshly ground black pepper

¼ cup nonfat plain Greek yogurt

1 tablespoon chopped fresh dill or ¼ teaspoon dried dill

1 tablespoon finely chopped scallion

2 (2-ounce) salmon fillets

½ teaspoon freshly squeezed lemon juice

1 tomato, cut into slices

1. Preheat the oven to 400°F. Line two baking sheets with nonstick aluminum foil.

2. Place the potato on the right side of one of the prepared baking sheets, drizzle with the oil, and season with garlic powder, salt, and pepper to taste. Fold the foil over the potato, pinching the edges to create a packet. Bake for 20 minutes.

3. Meanwhile, in a small bowl, stir together the yogurt, dill, and scallion. Season with salt and pepper to taste.

4. Place the salmon fillets on the right side of the second lined baking sheet. Drizzle the fish with the lemon juice; then spread the yogurt mix on top. Fold the foil over the salmon, pinching the edges to create a packet.

5. After the potato has been in the oven for 5 minutes, place the fish in the oven with the potatoes and bake for 15 minutes or until the fish flakes easily with a fork and the potato is soft. Transfer to a plate and garnish with tomato slices before serving.

PER SERVING *(4½ ounces)*: Protein: 16g; Calories: 144; Fat: 5g; Carbohydrates: 10g; Fiber: 1g; Total sugar: 4g; Added sugar: 0g; Sodium: 102mg

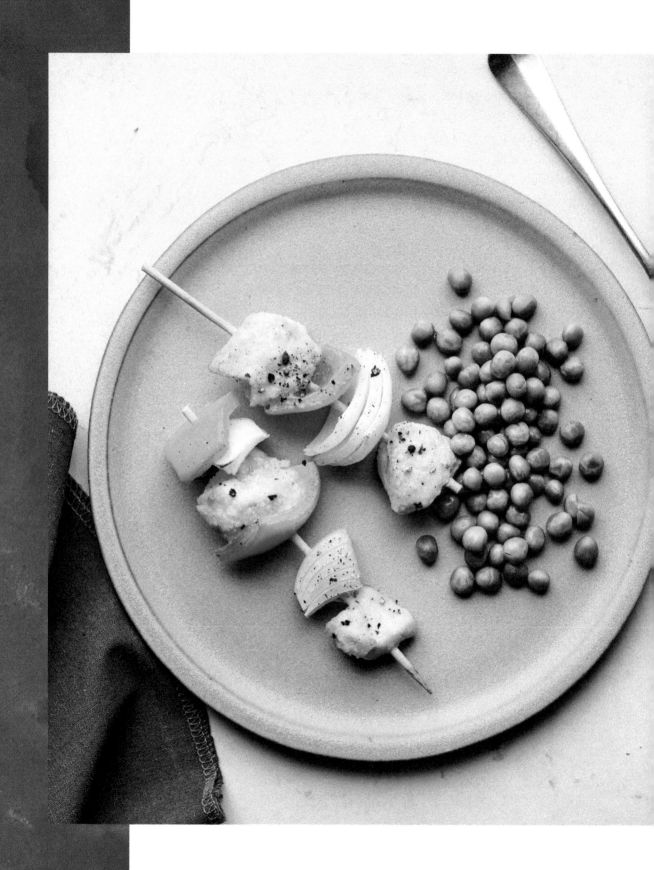

CHAPTER NINE

POULTRY

CHICKEN APPLE SALAD

SERVES 2 // **PREP TIME:** 15 minutes

This chicken salad is full of protein from the chicken and yogurt and fiber from the fruits and vegetables. Instead of cranberries, use raisins or diced grapes. Pair this salad with whole-grain toast or whole-grain crackers for a filling meal.

4 ounces cooked chicken breast, chopped

1 small apple, cored and diced

3 tablespoons nonfat plain Greek yogurt

2 tablespoons diced celery

2 teaspoons unsweetened dried cranberries

1 teaspoon chopped scallion or fresh chives

Salt

Freshly ground black pepper

Garlic powder, for seasoning

1. In a small bowl, stir together the chicken, apple, yogurt, celery, cranberries, and scallion.

2. Taste and season with salt, pepper, and garlic powder. Mix well.

STORAGE TIP: Refrigerate this salad in an airtight container for up to 2 days.

PER SERVING *(5 ounces)*: Protein: 18g; Calories: 142; Fat: 2g; Carbohydrates: 14g; Fiber: 2g; Total sugar: 10g; Added sugar: 0g; Sodium: 386mg

LAYERED MASON JAR CHICKEN SALAD

SERVES 1 // **PREP TIME**: 15 minutes

30 Minutes or Less
No Cook
One Pot

Salads made in a Mason jar not only are visually appealing but are easy to make ahead and take to work. Place hearty vegetables at the bottom, and then top with protein, a grain or starch, and greens. Olive oil with a little salt and pepper is an easy healthy dressing, but you may also try this salad with a variety of flavored olive oils or your favorite low-calorie dressing. Feel free to get creative.

¼ cup diced cucumber

¼ cup diced tomato

1 tablespoon diced bell pepper, red, orange, or yellow

2 ounces cooked chicken breast, diced

¼ cup Herb Quinoa (page 171)

½ cup shredded lettuce

2 teaspoons olive oil

Salt

Freshly ground black pepper

⅛ avocado, peeled, pitted, and diced (optional)

Fresh cilantro, for garnish (optional)

1. In a large Mason jar, layer the cucumber, tomato, and bell pepper.

2. Add the chicken and quinoa; top with the lettuce.

3. When ready to eat, sprinkle with the oil, replace the lid, and gently shake to coat all the ingredients. Pour the salad onto a plate or into a bowl and season with salt and pepper to taste.

4. Top with the avocado and cilantro (if using).

SERVING TIP: Add the oil just before eating. If you pack this for lunch, store the olive oil separately in a small lidded container.

PER SERVING *(6½ ounces)*: Protein: 19g; Calories: 266; Fat: 14g; Carbohydrates: 17g; Fiber: 3g; Total sugar: 5g; Added sugar: 0g; Sodium: 378mg

CHICKEN PESTO SALAD WRAP

SERVES 1 // **PREP TIME:** 15 minutes

30 Minutes or Less
No Cook
One Pot

Pesto gives this wrap its delicious salty flavor and creaminess. In fact, you may not need any more salt in this recipe. If you don't have tortillas on hand, serve the chicken pesto mixture with whole-grain crackers or on whole-grain bread. For something lighter, omit the tortilla. You can also use raisins in place of grapes. To save time, many grocery stores sell precooked chicken in the refrigerated or deli section.

2 ounces cooked chicken, diced

¼ cup diced celery

¼ cup seedless grapes, diced

2 tablespoons light mayonnaise

1 teaspoon basil pesto

Salt

Freshly ground black pepper

1 medium (8-inch) whole-grain tortilla

1. In a medium bowl, combine the chicken, celery, grapes, mayonnaise, and pesto. Season with salt and pepper to taste and mix well to combine.

2. Spoon the mixture into the tortilla, fold, and enjoy.

COOKING TIP: Prepare extra servings of the pesto chicken filling and refrigerate them in an airtight container for up to 3 days. Spoon the filling into the tortilla just before eating to prevent the tortilla from getting soggy.

PER SERVING *(5 ounces)*: Protein: 21g; Calories: 347; Fat: 14g; Carbohydrates: 37g; Fiber: 4g; Total sugar: 9g; Added sugar: 0g; Sodium: 735mg

MEDITERRANEAN CHICKEN WRAP

SERVES 1 // **PREP TIME:** 10 minutes

This wrap requires only a handful of ingredients that can probably be found in your refrigerator or pantry. I prefer using cooked chicken breast for this recipe, but you can use lunch meat or cold cuts that are natural with no added nitrates. For variety, add your favorite flavored hummus, like roasted garlic or red bell pepper, or a different cheese such as mozzarella. Try marinated mushrooms, too.

- 1 medium (8-inch) whole-grain tortilla
- 1 tablespoon hummus
- 1 ounce cooked chicken
- 1 ounce sliced provolone cheese
- 1 tablespoon sliced green or black olives
- 1 tablespoon chopped artichoke heart

1. Place the tortilla on a plate. Spread the hummus over it; then layer on the chicken, provolone cheese, olives, and artichoke heart.

2. Wrap and enjoy.

STORAGE TIP: To save time, prepare the ingredients ahead and refrigerate in separate containers until ready to assemble and eat.

PER SERVING *(4½ ounces)*: Protein: 21g; Calories: 338; Fat: 15g; Carbohydrates: 30g; Fiber: 6g; Total sugar: 2g; Added sugar: 0g; Sodium: 885mg

OVEN-ROASTED CHICKEN KEBABS

SERVES 4 // **PREP TIME:** 15 minutes // **COOK TIME:** 20 minutes

The best way to cook kebabs is on a grill—but that's not the only way. Try making this delicious meal in the oven and you will be pleasantly surprised. For best results, marinate the chicken breast in 1 tablespoon of freshly squeezed lemon juice, a dash of lemon pepper, and a dash of salt 2 hours before cooking. I recommend serving the kebabs hot with a side of steamed peas. You can also add zucchini or pineapple to the skewers with the chicken.

2 tablespoons olive oil

Salt

Freshly ground
black pepper

Garlic powder, for
seasoning

Onion powder, for
seasoning

1 (8-ounce) boneless,
skinless chicken breast,
cut into 1½-inch cubes

½ onion, cut into
1½-inch pieces

1 bell pepper, red,
orange, or yellow, cut
into 1½-inch pieces

1 cup peas, fresh or frozen

¼ cup water

1. Preheat the oven to 400°F. Line a baking sheet with aluminum foil.

2. In a small bowl, whisk the oil with salt, pepper, garlic powder, and onion powder to taste. Add the chicken and toss to coat.

3. Alternating ingredients, thread the seasoned chicken cubes, onion, and bell pepper onto 4 wooden or metal skewers. Place the skewers on the prepared baking sheet.

4. Bake for 10 to 15 minutes, or until the chicken reaches an internal temperature of 165°F and is no longer pink.

5. While the kebabs cook, in a small saucepan over high heat, combine the peas and water and bring to boil. Reduce the heat to medium, cover the pan, and cook for 3 to 4 minutes, or until soft. Drain. Alternatively, steam frozen peas in the microwave according to the package directions.

6. For crispier kebabs, place the baking sheet under the broiler and broil for 2 to 3 minutes, just until browned, if desired.

7. Serve 1 skewer with ¼ cup of peas.

COOKING TIP: If you use wooden skewers, soak them in warm water for 20 to 30 minutes before threading or place thin foil strips on their exposed edges to prevent burning. Don't have skewers? Try toothpicks.

STORAGE TIP: Refrigerate leftovers in an airtight container for up to 3 days.

PER SERVING (5 ounces): Protein: 15g; Calories: 167; Fat: 9g; Carbohydrates: 8g; Fiber: 3g; Total sugar: 4g; Added sugar: 0g; Sodium: 29mg

EASY TERIYAKI CHICKEN STIR-FRY

30 Minutes or Less
One Pot

SERVES 4 // **PREP TIME**: 10 minutes // **COOK TIME**: 20 minutes

This recipe sounds fancy although it is easy to make. I recommend using a frozen stir-fry vegetable mix; however, use any frozen or fresh vegetables you like. Add red bell pepper for extra color and crunch. Pair the stir-fry with Herb Quinoa (page 171) to make this meal complete. This recipe tastes best with sesame oil; however, you can use vegetable oil or olive oil if you prefer.

1 tablespoon sesame oil

1 (8-ounce) boneless, skinless chicken breast, cut into bite-size pieces

1 teaspoon soy sauce

1 cup frozen stir-fry vegetables

2 tablespoons teriyaki sauce

2 scallions, chopped

1 cup Herb Quinoa (page 171)

1 tablespoon sesame seeds (optional)

1. In a large skillet over medium-low heat, heat the oil. Add the chicken and soy sauce. Increase the heat to medium and cook for about 5 minutes until the chicken is golden and fully cooked through, stirring frequently.

2. Add the frozen vegetables, cover the skillet, and cook for 7 to 10 minutes, or until softened.

3. Add the teriyaki sauce and scallions and toss to coat. Simmer for 1 to 2 minutes more.

4. Plate ½ cup of the chicken mixture over ¼ cup of quinoa to serve. Sprinkle with sesame seeds (if using) and enjoy.

PER SERVING *(6 ounces)*: Protein: 16g; Calories: 197; Fat: 8g; Carbohydrates: 15g; Fiber: 2g; Total sugar: 4g; Added sugar: 0g; Sodium: 452mg

CREAMY CHICKEN AND MUSHROOMS

30 Minutes or Less
One Pot

SERVES 1 // **PREP TIME**: 10 minutes // **COOK TIME**: 15 minutes

This recipe is for mushroom lovers and requires little time for prep. If you do not have cooked chicken, use canned chicken. Thigh meat can be used, too. There's no need to add extra salt because marinated mushrooms and cheese contain salt. As this is a low-carb recipe, pair it with fruit or add ¼ cup of cooked potatoes to the mixture.

2 ounces cooked chicken breast, shredded

¼ cup marinated mushrooms

1 tablespoon nonfat plain Greek yogurt

1 tablespoon shredded Parmesan cheese

Garlic powder, for seasoning

Onion powder, for seasoning

Freshly ground black pepper

Fresh parsley or cilantro, for garnish

5 cucumber slices

1. Preheat the oven to 375°F.

2. In a small bowl, combine the chicken, mushrooms, yogurt, and Parmesan cheese. Season with garlic powder, onion powder, and pepper to taste. Mix well. Transfer the chicken mixture to a 6-ounce ramekin.

3. Bake for 10 to 12 minutes until the chicken is hot and the cheese is melted.

4. Garnish with parsley and serve with the cucumber slices on the side. Enjoy.

COOKING TIP: If you have time, it is much tastier to sauté 1 tablespoon of minced white onion and 3 to 4 slices of fresh mushroom until golden and add them to the mixture—but don't add too much oil.

PER SERVING *(5 ounces)*: Protein: 20g; Calories: 145; Fat: 5g; Carbohydrates: 5g; Fiber: 1g; Total sugar: 3g; Added sugar: 0g; Sodium: 591mg

ORANGE CHICKEN AND QUINOA

5 Ingredients or Fewer
30 Minutes or Less
One Pot

SERVES 2 // **PREP TIME:** 5 minutes // **COOK TIME:** 15 minutes

This juicy sweet-and-sour chicken is a great alternative to take-out with less fat, sugar, and carbs. This recipe calls for cooked quinoa, which you can make a big batch of in advance (see Herb Quinoa, page 171). Keep refrigerated to serve alongside lunch or dinner, or buy it precooked and frozen to heat quickly in the microwave.

1 teaspoon vegetable oil

4 ounces boneless, skinless chicken breast, cut into 1-inch cubes

1 small orange, halved

Salt

¼ cup cooked quinoa

1. In a medium skillet over medium heat, heat the oil. Add the chicken to the skillet.

2. Thinly slice half of the orange and place the slices on the chicken. Squeeze the juice of the remaining half into the skillet to coat the chicken.

3. Cover the skillet and cook for 10 to 15 minutes, stirring occasionally, until the chicken is fully cooked with no pink remaining.

4. Season with salt to taste, stir to incorporate, and remove the skillet from the heat. Serve the chicken with the orange slices and a side of quinoa.

COOKING TIP: You can marinate the chicken with the orange slices and juice overnight, which will make the chicken even juicier and more tender. I recommend doubling this recipe: This chicken can be used as protein in salads and wraps or eaten warm with vegetables or any healthy grain.

PER SERVING *(4½ ounces)*: Protein: 17g; Calories: 158; Fat: 4g; Carbohydrates: 13g; Fiber: 2g; Total sugar: 6g; Added sugar: 0g; Sodium: 373mg

BAKED CHICKEN QUESADILLA AND VEGETABLES

SERVES 1 // **PREP TIME**: 10 minutes // **COOK TIME**: 10 minutes

A quesadilla is typically fried, but baking this iconic meal is easy and avoids unwanted fat and calories. Feel free to get creative: Use a different cheese, or swap black beans for corn or cooked ground turkey or chicken for more protein.

1 medium (8-inch) whole-grain tortilla

Olive oil, for brushing

1 ounce shredded pepper Jack cheese

1 ounce shredded cooked chicken

1 tablespoon diced bell pepper, red, orange, or yellow

1 tablespoon canned corn, drained and rinsed

1 tablespoon salsa or pico de gallo

⅛ avocado, peeled, pitted, and cut into slices (optional)

1. Preheat the oven to 400°F.

2. Place the tortilla on a baking sheet. Brush it with oil and flip it over.

3. Fill half the tortilla with pepper Jack cheese, chicken, bell pepper, and corn. Fold the empty half over to form a quesadilla.

4. Bake for 10 minutes. Serve with the salsa and avocado (if using).

COOKING TIP: For this recipe, prepare the ingredients ahead and refrigerate in separate containers. When ready to eat, just assemble the quesadilla and bake.

PER SERVING *(5 ounces)*: Protein: 19g; Calories: 304; Fat: 12g; Carbohydrates: 29g; Fiber: 4g; Total sugar: 3g; Added sugar: 0g; Sodium: 743mg

LEMON-PEPPER CHICKEN AND VEGETABLES

30 Minutes or Less
One Pot

SERVES 2 // **PREP TIME:** 10 minutes // **COOK TIME:** 20 minutes

I recommend keeping frozen vegetables on hand for quick, easy, healthy sides. For this recipe, I use a carrot, cauliflower, and broccoli blend, which you can find in the frozen section of most grocery stores. This recipe calls for a side of Herb Quinoa (page 171), which you can make a big batch of in advance. Keep refrigerated to serve alongside lunch or dinner during the week, or buy frozen cooked quinoa and heat it quickly in the microwave. You can also pair the chicken and vegetables with any grain you have on hand.

Olive oil spray (optional)

4 ounces boneless, skinless chicken breast, cut into 1-inch cubes

1 teaspoon freshly squeezed lemon juice

Lemon pepper, for seasoning

Salt

½ cup frozen mixed vegetables

1 teaspoon olive oil

½ cup Herb Quinoa (page 171)

1. Preheat the oven to 400°F. Coat a 9-by-5-inch baking dish with olive oil spray, or line it with nonstick aluminum foil.

2. Place the chicken into the prepared baking dish. Drizzle it with lemon juice and season with lemon pepper and salt to taste.

3. Bake for 10 to 15 minutes until the chicken is fully cooked with no pink remaining.

4. While the chicken bakes, steam the frozen vegetables in the microwave according to the package directions. Drizzle the cooked vegetables with the oil.

5. Serve 2 ounces of chicken with ¼ cup of vegetables and ¼ cup of herb quinoa. Enjoy.

COOKING TIP: This chicken will taste even better and be more tender if you marinate it in the lemon juice and spices for several hours in the refrigerator before baking.

PER SERVING *(5 ounces)*: Protein: 19g; Calories: 217; Fat: 7g; Carbohydrates: 19g; Fiber: 3g; Total sugar: 4g; Added sugar: 0g; Sodium: 379mg

BASIL PESTO CHICKEN AND BRUSSELS SPROUTS

30 Minutes or Less

SERVES 3 // **PREP TIME**: 10 minutes // **COOK TIME**: 20 minutes

Brussels sprouts are among the healthiest foods because they are low in calories and high in fiber. This recipe calls for a side of quinoa (see Herb Quinoa, page 171); you can make a big batch of it in advance and keep it refrigerated to serve alongside lunch or dinner during the week or buy it frozen and heat it quickly in the microwave. If you don't like quinoa, this meal is great with brown rice or risotto.

¾ cup thinly sliced Brussels sprouts

1 tablespoon olive oil

6 ounces boneless, skinless chicken breast

3 teaspoons basil pesto

1 tablespoon shredded Parmesan cheese

Balsamic glaze, for drizzling

¾ cup cooked quinoa

1. Preheat the oven to 425°F. Line two baking sheets with aluminum foil.

2. Place the Brussels sprouts on one of the prepared baking sheets and drizzle with the oil.

3. Cut the chicken into 3 thin slices and place them on the second baking sheet. Spoon 1 teaspoon of pesto onto each piece of chicken and wrap the foil over the chicken, pinching the edges to create a packet.

4. Place the baking sheets on different oven racks and cook for 15 to 20 minutes, or until the chicken is fully cooked with no pink remaining.

5. When the Brussels sprouts are done (they should be soft with browned edges), remove them from the oven, sprinkle with the Parmesan cheese, and drizzle with balsamic glaze.

6. Serve 2 ounces of chicken with ¼ cup of Brussels sprouts and ¼ cup of quinoa and enjoy.

STORAGE TIP: Refrigerate extra portions in an airtight container for up to 3 days and reheat when ready to eat.

PER SERVING *(6 ounces)*: Protein: 16g; Calories: 198; Fat: 10g; Carbohydrates: 12g; Fiber: 2g; Sugar: 1g; Added sugar: 0g; Sodium: 113mg

JUICY CHICKEN PATTIES WITH GARLIC CAULIFLOWER AND POTATO MASH

5 Ingredients or Fewer
30 Minutes or Less

SERVES 8 // **PREP TIME**: 10 minutes // **COOK TIME**: 15 minutes

I never buy premade patties because homemade patties are juicier and taste better and you know what is in them. To change up the flavor of these patties, experiment with your favorite dried herbs, such as basil, dill, or rosemary, or use lean ground beef or turkey. The trick to keeping the patties moist is adding water to the pan. I pair the patties with Garlic Cauliflower and Potato Mash (page 172), but serve them with your favorite grain or vegetables as desired.

1 pound ground chicken

1 large egg

2 garlic cloves, minced

Onion powder, for
    seasoning

Salt

Freshly ground
    black pepper

1 tablespoon olive oil

¼ cup water

4 cups Garlic Cauliflower
    and Potato Mash
    (page 172)

1. In a medium bowl, combine the ground chicken, egg, and garlic. Season with onion powder, salt, and pepper to taste. Mix well. Divide the meat mixture into 8 portions (2 ounces each). Roll each into a ball, and then form into a patty.

2. In a large skillet over medium heat, heat the oil. Add the water; then place the chicken patties in the skillet and cover the skillet with a lid. Cook for 7 minutes, flip, and cook for 7 minutes more until fully cooked with no pink remaining.

3. Remove from the heat and serve each patty with ½ cup of cauliflower-potato mash. Enjoy.

STORAGE TIP: This recipe makes 8 patties. Refrigerate extras in an airtight container or zip-top plastic bag for up to 3 days. Or freeze in a freezer-safe plastic zip-top bag, tightly sealed with as much air as possible pressed out, for up to 6 months.

SERVING TIP: These patties pair well with salads or can be used as the filling for a wrap with vegetables.

PER SERVING *(5½ ounces)*: Protein: 16g; Calories: 259; Fat: 12g; Carbohydrates: 23g; Fiber: 3g; Total sugar: 2g; Added sugar: 0g; Sodium: 134mg

THANKSGIVING-INSPIRED TURKEY WRAP

5 Ingredients or Fewer
30 Minutes or Less
No Cook
One Pot

SERVES 1 // **PREP TIME:** 10 minutes

The secret ingredient in this recipe is the sweet and sour cranberry. If you find orange-flavored dried cranberries, those are a great option for this dish, too. I highly recommend making this wrap with real turkey instead of deli meat because it is lower in fat and sodium and does not have added nitrates or preservatives.

1 medium (8-inch) whole-grain tortilla

1 tablespoon light cream cheese

1 tablespoon dried cranberries

2 ounces sliced cooked turkey breast

1. Place the tortilla on a plate and spread the cream cheese over it. Sprinkle on the cranberries and top with the turkey.

2. Wrap tightly and enjoy immediately.

PER SERVING *(4½ ounces)*: Protein: 14g; Calories: 260; Fat: 8g; Carbohydrates: 35g; Fiber: 4g; Total sugar: 9g; Added sugar: 0g; Sodium: 861mg

PARMESAN-OAT TURKEY BURGERS

30 Minutes or Less

SERVES 8 // **PREP TIME**: 10 minutes // **COOK TIME**: 20 minutes

This turkey burger with rolled oats is soft, tender, and incredibly juicy, thanks to the water added to the pan during cooking. Change up the flavors by adding herbs, such as basil, cilantro, or dill. Because this is a low-carbohydrate recipe, you can pair it with fruit or serve it on a whole-grain bun or with a side of your favorite grain or steamed vegetables. This burger is delicious topped with provolone cheese, but Gouda or white Cheddar also works well.

1 pound lean
  ground turkey

1 large egg

½ cup rolled oats

½ cup shredded
  Parmesan cheese

2 tablespoons
  Worcestershire sauce

1 tablespoon
  dried parsley

Salt

Freshly ground
  black pepper

Onion powder, for
  seasoning

1 tablespoon olive oil

¼ cup water

8 slices (1 ounce)
  provolone cheese

8 romaine lettuce leaves
  or butter lettuce leaves

1. In a medium bowl, combine the ground turkey, egg, oats, Parmesan cheese, Worcestershire sauce, and parsley. Season with salt, pepper, and onion powder to taste. Mix well.

2. Divide the meat mixture into 8 portions (2 ounces each). Roll each into a ball, and then form into a patty.

3. In a large skillet over medium heat, heat the oil. Add the water; then place the turkey patties into the skillet and cover the skillet with a lid. Cook for 5 to 7 minutes, flip, and cook for 5 to 7 minutes more until the meat is fully cooked with no pink remaining.

4. Transfer any patties not needed for this meal to a plate to cool before refrigerating for future use.

5. Top each remaining patty in the skillet with 1 slice of provolone cheese. Cover the skillet and cook for 2 to 3 minutes, or until the cheese melts. Serve each patty on a lettuce leaf.

COOKING TIP: You can also bake the turkey mixture in a baking dish (like a meatloaf), in 6-ounce ramekins, or in a muffin tin. Bake in a 400°F oven for about 15 minutes until fully cooked with no pink remaining.

STORAGE TIP: Refrigerate leftover cooked patties in an airtight container for up to 3 days, or freeze for up to 6 months. Add the cheese after reheating the patty.

PER SERVING *(2-ounce burger)*: Protein: 22g; Calories: 266; Fat: 17g; Carbohydrates: 6g; Fiber: 1g; Total sugar: 1g; Added sugar: 0g; Sodium: 402mg

COLORFUL TURKEY MEATLOAF

SERVES 8 // **PREP TIME:** 15 minutes // **COOK TIME:** 25 minutes

Meatloaf is a classic comfort food that can also be nutritious and healthy. This hearty meatloaf is juicy and full of goodness—sweetness from the bell pepper and carrot and a punch of flavor from the garlic and herbs. Choose sweet bell peppers like red, orange, or yellow. You can pair the meatloaf with Garlic Cauliflower and Potato Mash (page 172) as here or your favorite grain or potatoes. Instead of turkey, use ground chicken or lean ground beef. Instead of parsley, try dill or mix parsley and dill together.

Nonstick cooking spray

1 pound ground turkey

½ cup diced carrot

½ cup diced bell pepper, red, orange, or yellow

3 garlic cloves, minced

1 teaspoon onion powder

½ teaspoon dried parsley

Freshly ground black pepper

Salt

3 tablespoons shredded low-fat Cheddar cheese

4 cups Garlic Cauliflower and Potato Mash (page 172)

1. Preheat the oven to 425°F. Coat a 10-by-5-inch glass baking dish with cooking spray.

2. In a medium bowl, combine the ground turkey, carrot, bell pepper, garlic, onion powder, and parsley. Season with pepper and salt to taste. Mix well. Transfer the meatloaf mixture to the prepared baking dish, spreading it into an even layer, and cover the dish with aluminum foil.

3. Bake for 15 to 20 minutes until fully cooked with no pink remaining. Uncover the meatloaf and sprinkle it with the Cheddar cheese. Bake, uncovered for 5 minutes more, or until the cheese melts.

4. Let the meatloaf cool slightly before serving. Serve 3 ounces of meatloaf (one-eighth of the loaf) with ½ cup of cauliflower-potato mash. Enjoy.

COOKING TIP: Use a muffin tin to bake mini meatloaves, or bake in individual 6-ounce ramekins. Reduce the baking time to 10 to 15 minutes.

STORAGE TIP: Refrigerate leftover meatloaf in an airtight container for up to 3 days, or freeze for up to 6 months.

PER SERVING *(6 ½ ounces)*: Protein: 16g; Calories: 264; Fat: 12g; Carbohydrates: 25g; Fiber: 3g; Total sugar: 3g; Added sugar: 0g; Sodium: 103mg

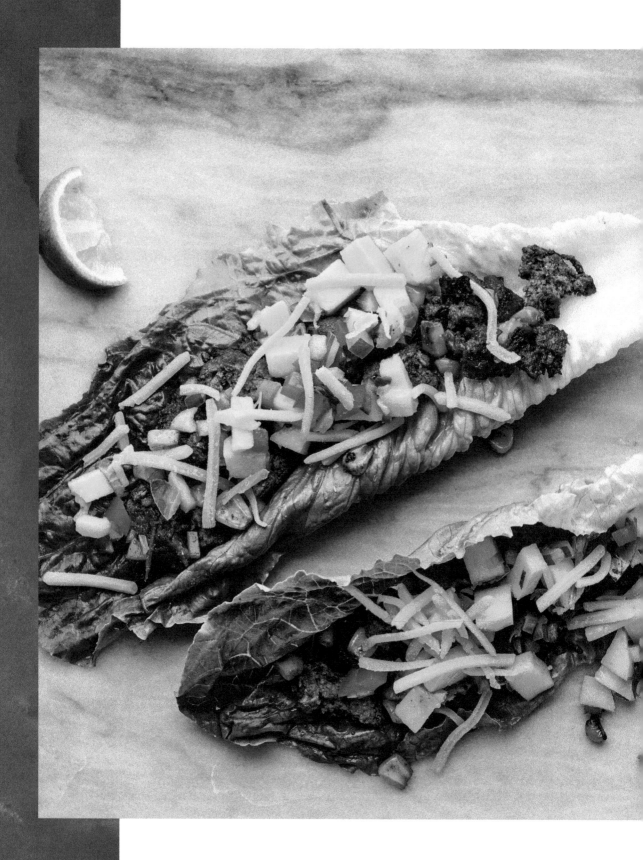

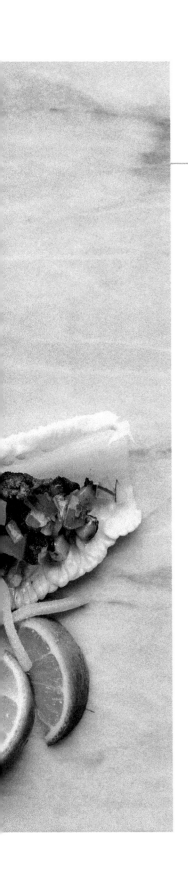

CHAPTER TEN

PORK AND BEEF

MINI HAM AND LETTUCE SALAD

SERVES 2 // **PREP TIME:** 15 minutes // **COOK TIME:** 15 minutes

This salad has protein, fiber, and carbohydrates—a complete meal in minutes. I like having frozen peas on hand, as canned peas can be mushy. Choose a precooked ham that's uncured with no added nitrates.

1 carrot

⅓ cup frozen peas

⅓ cup canned corn, drained and rinsed

4 ounces diced cooked ham

3 tablespoons light mayonnaise

Dried dill, for seasoning (optional)

4 iceberg lettuce leaves

1. In a medium saucepan over high heat, combine the carrot and 2 to 3 inches of water to cover. Bring to a boil and cook for 10 to 15 minutes until the carrot is soft. Let the carrot cool; then peel and dice it.

2. Pour the peas into a small bowl and let thaw, or put them in a small microwave-safe bowl and microwave on high power for 1 minute or until thawed. Drain the water.

3. Add the diced carrot to the peas along with the corn, ham, and mayonnaise. Season with dill to taste (if using). Mix well. Divide the salad among the lettuce leaves and enjoy.

STORAGE TIP: Refrigerate this salad in an airtight container for up to 3 days. Spoon into the lettuce leaves just before serving.

PER SERVING *(2 filled lettuce leaves; 5 ounces)*: Calories: 173; Protein: 11g; Fat: 8g; Carbohydrates: 15g; Fiber: 3g; Total sugar: 7g; Added sugar: 0g; Sodium: 1017mg

HAM, POTATO, AND ONION STACK

30 Minutes or Less
One Pot

SERVES 2 // **PREP TIME**: 10 minutes // **COOK TIME**: 20 minutes

This is a very easy recipe to make at home—especially if you're a meat and potato lover. I prefer Canadian bacon because it has great flavor and the meat is thick. When you buy ham or Canadian bacon, choose only uncured meats with no nitrates added. The light mayonnaise on top of the cheese prevents the cheese from burning. Instead of Cheddar, try pepper Jack cheese.

Olive oil spray

½ russet potato

4 ounces Canadian bacon, thinly sliced into 4 pieces

½ white onion, thinly sliced into rings

4 tablespoons shredded low-fat Cheddar cheese

4 teaspoons light mayonnaise

Freshly ground black pepper

1 tomato, cut into slices

1. Preheat the oven to 400°F. Line a baking sheet with aluminum foil and spray it with olive oil spray.

2. Peel the potato and cut it into 4 thin, round slices, about ¼ inch thick. Place the potato slices on the prepared baking sheet and layer each with 1 slice of Canadian bacon, some onion rings, and 1 tablespoon of Cheddar cheese. Spread 1 teaspoon of mayonnaise on top.

3. Bake for 15 to 20 minutes, or until the potatoes are soft and golden brown.

4. Season with pepper to taste and garnish with tomato slices to serve. Enjoy warm.

COOKING TIP: To add flavor, sprinkle on fresh or dried herbs, such as cilantro, dill, or parsley, before baking. If you keep fresh herbs on hand, to keep them from going bad, chop the herbs and freeze them in a glass jar for up to 3 months.

PER SERVING *(4 ounces)*: Calories: 226; Protein: 22g; Fat: 5g; Carbohydrates: 24g; Fiber: 2g; Total sugar: 4g; Added sugar: 0g; Sodium: 782mg

SAUERKRAUT BAKED PORK CHOPS

SERVES 2 // **PREP TIME**: 10 minutes // **COOK TIME**: 20 minutes

Sauerkraut is fermented cabbage. It is a superfood because it has fiber, vitamin C, and beneficial probiotics (good bacteria) produced during the fermentation process. To make sure you're using a sauerkraut with probiotic properties, choose one without vinegar in the ingredients. There's no need to add salt to this recipe, as sauerkraut is salty. Slice the pork chops thinly so they will cook faster. This recipe pairs well with freshly sliced tomato and cucumber.

Olive oil, for greasing

2 (2-ounce) lean boneless pork chops, cut into ½-inch cubes

Freshly ground black pepper

1 russet potato, cut into ½-inch cubes

½ cup drained sauerkraut

4 tablespoons water or vegetable broth

1. Preheat the oven to 400°F. Coat 2 (6-ounce) ramekins with oil.

2. Evenly divide the pork between the prepared ramekins. Season with pepper to taste.

3. Top the pork in each ramekin with half the potato cubes and then ¼ cup of sauerkraut.

4. Pour 2 tablespoons of water into each ramekin. Cover the ramekins with aluminum foil.

5. Bake for 15 to 20 minutes, or until the internal temperature reaches 145°F and the meat is white, not pink. Enjoy warm.

COOKING TIP: Swap sauerkraut for very thinly chopped fresh cabbage.

PER SERVING (5 ounces): Calories: 165; Protein: 15g; Fat: 2g; Carbohydrates: 21g; Fiber: 4g; Total sugar: 2g; Added sugar: 0g; Sodium: 424mg

BARBECUE PORK PATTIES WITH SWEET POTATOES

30 Minutes or Less

SERVES 4 // **PREP TIME:** 10 minutes // **COOK TIME:** 20 minutes

This recipe is for people who love meat and potatoes. I use lean pork here, but you can also combine lean pork and beef. Choose your favorite barbecue sauce, preferably one that is low in sugar. You can serve this meal with a fresh vegetable salad on the side.

Olive oil spray (optional)

1 sweet potato, cut into 1-inch cubes

8 ounces lean ground pork

1 large egg

¼ cup minced white onion

2 garlic cloves, minced

½ teaspoon salt

½ teaspoon freshly ground black pepper

1 tablespoon olive oil

½ cup water

4 tablespoons barbecue sauce

1. Preheat the oven to 400°F. Line a baking sheet with nonstick aluminum foil, or spray the sheet with olive oil spray.

2. Place the sweet potato on the baking sheet and bake for 20 minutes, or until soft.

3. Meanwhile, in a small bowl, mix the ground pork, egg, onion, garlic, salt, and pepper. Divide the meat mixture into 4 portions (2 ounces each). Roll each into a ball, and then flatten into a ½-inch-thick patty.

4. In a skillet over medium heat, heat the oil. Add the patties to the skillet and cook for 2 minutes per side.

5. Add the water to the skillet, cover, and reduce the heat to medium-low. Simmer for 5 to 7 minutes, flip, re-cover, and simmer for 5 to 7 minutes more until cooked through and no longer pink.

6. Plate the patties, top each with 1 tablespoon of barbecue sauce, and serve with ¼ cup of sweet potato.

PER SERVING *(4 ounces)*: Protein: 14g; Calories: 179; Fat: 7g; Carbohydrates: 15g; Fiber: 1g; Total sugar: 7g; Added sugar: 0g; Sodium: 564mg

MEAT LOVER'S CHILI BOWL

One Pot

SERVES 8 // **PREP TIME:** 20 minutes // **COOK TIME:** 35 minutes

Slightly smoky and sweet, this chili is hard to resist with its scent of cumin, savory tomatoes, and just a touch of chili spice. You can use your favorite chili seasoning mix instead of the spices listed here or add cayenne pepper. I like to serve my chili bowl topped with a teaspoon of Greek yogurt, shredded cheese, and black olives. Use canned black beans or red kidney beans in this recipe if preferred.

1 tablespoon olive oil

½ cup diced white onion

2 garlic cloves, minced

1 pound lean ground beef

1 (15-ounce) can diced tomatoes, with their juices

1 (15-ounce) can white chili beans, with their juices

½ cup canned corn, drained and rinsed

1 tablespoon chili powder

½ teaspoon ground cumin

Salt

8 tablespoons nonfat plain Greek yogurt (optional)

8 tablespoons shredded low-fat Cheddar cheese (optional)

1. In a large pot over medium heat, heat the oil. Add the onion and garlic and sauté for about 5 minutes until light golden brown.

2. Add the ground beef and cook, stirring to break up the meat into smaller chunks, for 5 to 10 minutes, or until browned.

3. Add the tomatoes with their juices, chili beans with their juices, corn, chili powder, and cumin. Season with salt to taste and stir to combine. Reduce the heat to low, cover the pot, and simmer the chili for about 15 minutes.

4. Serve warm, topping each portion with 1 tablespoon of yogurt (if using) and 1 tablespoon of Cheddar cheese (if using). Enjoy.

COOKING TIP: You can swap ground beef for lean ground turkey or chicken.

PER SERVING *(6½ ounces)*: Protein: 19g; Calories: 210; Fat: 7g; Carbohydrates: 16g; Fiber: 5g; Total sugar: 4g; Added sugar: 0g; Sodium: 478mg

BAKED BASIL MEATBALLS

30 Minutes or Less

SERVES 4 // **PREP TIME:** 10 minutes // **COOK TIME:** 15 minutes

These meatballs are high in protein, take little time to make, and will fill your kitchen with the fragrant scent of fresh basil. Here, I pair the meatballs with spiralized carrot, but you can use any vegetable. You can usually find spiralized vegetables in the refrigerated area of your grocery store's fresh produce section. A julienne peeler also does the trick.

8 ounces lean ground beef

1 large egg

2 garlic cloves, minced

¼ cup minced red onion

¼ cup chopped fresh basil leaves

¼ cup shredded or grated Parmesan cheese

2 tablespoons nonfat milk

12 ounces spiralized carrot, fresh or frozen

Salt

Freshly ground black pepper

1 teaspoon olive oil

1. Preheat the oven to 415°F. Line a large baking sheet with aluminum foil. Set aside.

2. In a medium bowl, combine the ground beef, egg, garlic, red onion, basil, Parmesan cheese, and milk. Mix the ingredients until well combined. Form the mixture into about 8 small (1-tablespoon) balls and place them on the prepared baking sheet about ½ inch apart.

3. Bake for 10 to 15 minutes until browned and no longer pink in the middle and the meatballs reach an internal temperature of 160°F.

4. While the meatballs bake, bring a medium pot of water to a boil over high heat. Add the carrot and cook for 2 to 4. Drain. Season the carrot with salt and pepper to taste and drizzle with the oil.

5. Serve 2 meatballs with ½ cup of spiralized carrot and enjoy.

COOKING TIP: Use lean ground turkey if you prefer. Also, use ½ teaspoon of dried basil instead of fresh.

PER SERVING *(4 ounces)*: Protein: 20g; Calories: 197; Fat: 9g; Carbohydrates: 9g; Fiber: 3g; Total sugar: 4g; Added sugar: 0g; Sodium: 186mg

UNSTUFFED BELL PEPPERS

5 Ingredients or Fewer
One Pot

SERVES 2 // **PREP TIME**: 10 minutes // **COOK TIME**: 30 minutes

Stuffed vegetables, in this case bell peppers, have been popular for many years around the world, and for good reason—they're insanely delicious. This particular recipe was simplified to be a "lazy" version featuring lean ground beef, aromatic vegetables, and spices. You can use a variety of tomato sauces: garlic, marinara, or basil. To save time, buy diced fresh vegetables in the refrigerated area of your grocer's produce section. I suggest using red, orange, or yellow bell peppers or sweet mini bell peppers for this recipe.

1 tablespoon olive oil

¼ cup diced onion

⅓ cup shredded carrot

4 ounces lean
    ground beef

Salt

Freshly ground
    black pepper

½ cup diced bell pepper,
    red, yellow, or orange

½ cup favorite mari-
    nara sauce

Nonfat plain Greek
    yogurt, for serving
    (optional)

1. In a small pan over medium heat, heat the oil. Add the onion and carrot and sauté for 5 to 7 minutes until softened.

2. Add the ground beef and season with salt and pepper to taste. Cook for 5 to 7 minutes, breaking up the meat with a spatula.

3. Add the bell pepper and cook for 5 minutes more.

4. Stir in the marinara sauce. Cover the pan with a lid, reduce the heat to low, and simmer for 5 to 10 minutes.

5. Divide between 2 bowls, top each with a dollop of yogurt (if using), and enjoy. Refrigerate leftovers for up to 3 days.

COOKING TIP: Any lean ground meat can be used in this recipe.

PER SERVING *(6½ ounces)*: Protein: 17g; Calories: 235; Fat: 13g; Carbohydrates: 13g; Fiber: 3g; Total sugar: 8g; Added sugar: 0g; Sodium: 282mg

JUICY BUN-LESS BEEF BURGERS

SERVES 4 // **PREP TIME**: 10 minutes // **COOK TIME**: 16 minutes

This is one of the easiest and fastest ways to cook a burger. To keep this dish low-carb, serve the burger on a lettuce leaf, if desired. Use leftover cooked burger patties as the filling for wraps and tacos.

1 teaspoon olive oil, plus more for preparing the ramekins

8 ounces lean ground beef

2 teaspoons Worcester-shire sauce

Salt

Freshly ground black pepper

4 slices low-fat Cheddar cheese or other low-fat cheese

4 onion slices, diced

4 tomato slices, cubed

2 cups Garlic Cauliflower and Potato Mash (page 172)

1. Preheat the oven to 420°F. Coat 4 (6-ounce) ramekins with oil and set aside.

2. In a medium bowl, combine the oil, beef, and Worcestershire sauce. Season with salt and pepper and mix well to combine. Evenly divide the mixture among the prepared ramekins and press into a burger shape.

3. Bake for 10 to 13 minutes, or until cooked through and no longer pink.

4. Remove the ramekins from the oven and top each burger with 1 slice of cheese. Bake for 2 to 3 minutes more to melt the cheese.

5. Remove the ramekins from the oven. Transfer the burgers to plates—or keep them in the ramekins—and top each with onion and tomato. Serve each burger with ½ cup of cauliflower-potato mash and enjoy.

STORAGE TIP: Refrigerate the burgers, cooked or raw, in an airtight container or in tightly covered ramekins in the refrigerator for up to 3 days, or freeze for up to 6 months.

COOKING TIP: Top with pickled red onions (see Cooking Tip, page 157).

PER SERVING *(5 ounces)*: Protein: 26g; Calories: 343; Fat: 15g; Carbohydrates: 26g; Fiber: 3g; Total sugar: 4g; Added sugar: 0g; Sodium: 344mg

TORTILLA-LESS MINI BEEF TACOS

30 Minutes or Less
One Pot

SERVES 2 // **PREP TIME**: 15 minutes // **COOK TIME**: 15 minutes

Romaine lettuce can be a great low-carb, less-filling alternative to tortillas for taco lovers. I highly recommend serving this recipe with my sweetly refreshing Mango Salsa (page 168); however, regular salsa is also delicious.

1½ teaspoons olive oil

4 ounces lean ground beef

¼ teaspoon taco seasoning

2 tablespoons canned no-salt-added diced tomatoes, drained

2 tablespoons corn kernels, frozen or canned and drained

2 romaine lettuce leaves

2 tablespoons Mango Salsa (page 168)

1 tablespoon shredded low-fat Cheddar cheese

1 lime, cut into wedges (optional)

1. In a large skillet over medium heat, heat the oil. Add the ground beef and taco seasoning. Cook for about 5 minutes, stirring to break up the meat into smaller chunks.

2. Stir in the tomatoes and corn. Reduce the heat to low, cover the skillet, and simmer for about 5 minutes, stirring occasionally. Remove the skillet from the heat.

3. Place the lettuce leaves on a plate. Fill each with beef mixture and top each serving with 1 tablespoon of mango salsa and ½ tablespoon of Cheddar cheese.

4. Serve with lime wedges (if using) and enjoy.

COOKING TIP: For a touch of spice, top with a dash of your favorite hot sauce.

PER SERVING *(3½ ounces)*: Protein: 17g; Calories: 178; Fat: 9g; Carbohydrates: 8g; Fiber: 2g; Total sugar: 4g; Added sugar: 0g; Sodium: 96mg

BEEF WRAP WITH HORSERADISH AND PICKLED ONIONS

30 Minutes or Less
No Cook
One Pot

SERVES 1 // **PREP TIME**: 15 minutes

This is an easy, flavorful recipe for those meals when you just don't have time to cook but still want something filling, packed with protein and veggies. If you don't have lettuce, use spinach or arugula. Pita can work in place of a tortilla. When shopping for sliced beef, choose a deli meat with no added nitrates.

1 medium (8-inch) whole-grain tortilla

2 teaspoons horseradish sauce

2 ounces sliced cooked beef

Worcestershire sauce, for seasoning

1½ tablespoons pickled onion (see Cooking Tip)

4 slices cucumber

2 slices tomato

¼ cup shredded lettuce

⅛ avocado, peeled, pitted, and cut into slices (optional)

1. Place the tortilla on a plate and spread the horseradish over it.

2. Add the beef slices and a dash of Worcestershire sauce to taste.

3. Layer on the pickled onion, cucumber, tomato, lettuce, and avocado (if using). Tightly wrap and enjoy.

STORAGE TIP: Prep all the ingredients ahead and refrigerate them in separate containers. Just assemble the wrap when ready to eat.

COOKING TIP: Pickled onions are a great addition to any sandwich, salad, wrap, or burger. You can find them in the canned vegetable aisle—or you can make your own. In a small bowl, combine 1 cup of water, ½ cup of white vinegar, 1 tablespoon of sugar, and 1½ teaspoons of salt. Stir until dissolved. In a glass jar, combine 1 red onion, thinly sliced, and 5 to 8 peppercorns. Pour the vinegar mixture over the top. Add 1 garlic clove, minced, if you like. Let sit at room temperature for 1 hour; then cover and refrigerate for 2 to 3 months. Drain the brine before serving the pickled onion slices.

PER SERVING *(4½ ounces)*: Protein: 16g; Calories: 275; Fat: 11g; Carbohydrates: 30g; Fiber: 5g; Total sugar: 4g; Added sugar: 0g; Sodium: 884mg

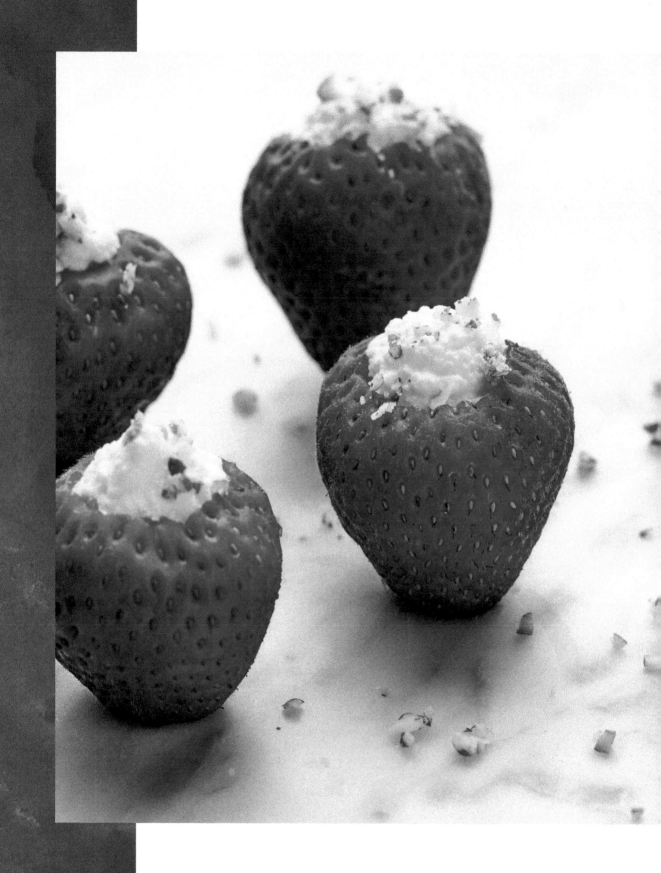

CHAPTER ELEVEN

DESSERT

JUICY PEACH DESSERT

SERVES 1 // **PREP TIME:** 10 minutes

This is one of my favorite desserts. It is low-calorie, mouthwatering, and easy to make. Plus, it contains fiber, protein, and natural sugars from the fruit, honey, and yogurt. It also makes a satisfying snack between meals.

1 peach, halved and pitted

4 tablespoons nonfat plain Greek yogurt

1 teaspoon ground cinnamon

1 teaspoon honey

1. Place the peach halves on a plate. Spoon 2 tablespoons of Greek yogurt into each cavity left by the pit.

2. Sprinkle with cinnamon, drizzle with honey, and enjoy.

COOKING TIP: Warm peaches taste even more delicious. Microwave the peach halves on high power for 30 to 60 seconds, or place them in a skillet over low heat, cut-side down, and cook for 1 to 2 minutes—before adding the toppings. For fewer calories and more flavor options, use any sugar-free syrup you prefer instead of honey. If you can't find fresh peaches, use no-sugar-added canned peaches.

POST-OP TIP: In the first few weeks following surgery, start with ½ peach for dessert.

PER SERVING (*4 ounces*): Protein: 8g; Calories: 123; Fat: 1g; Carbohydrates: 24g; Fiber: 4g; Total sugar: 20g; Added sugar: 6g; Sodium: 23mg

CRUSTLESS APPLE PIE WITH NUT BUTTER

5 Ingredients or Fewer
One Pot

SERVES 1 // **PREP TIME**: 10 minutes // **COOK TIME**: 20 to 30 minutes

If you love apples as much as I do, this recipe is pure joy. You can enjoy this delicious dessert warm or cold and even make variations by changing the type of nut or seed butter, swapping raisins for cranberries, and so on. It's also delicious paired with 1 tablespoon of sugar-free ice cream.

1 small apple or ½ medium apple, cored

1 tablespoon almond butter

7 raisins, no added sugar

1 teaspoon shredded unsweetened coconut

Ground cinnamon, for seasoning

Sugar-free syrup or honey, for drizzling (optional)

1 pecan, chopped (optional)

1. Preheat the oven to 375°F.

2. Cut the apple into thin slices or wedges or small pieces the size of a dime.

3. In a medium bowl, stir together the apple, almond butter, raisins, and coconut. Sprinkle with cinnamon to taste. Mix well so the nut butter coats everything. Transfer the mixture to a 6-ounce ramekin or small baking dish.

4. Bake for 20 to 30 minutes until the apple is tender. If you like apples crispy, bake for less time (closer to 20 minutes).

5. Remove from the oven and drizzle with syrup (if using). Top with the pecan (if using) and enjoy.

STORAGE TIP: Make several ramekins of this apple pie at one time and refrigerate them, covered with plastic wrap or in an airtight container, for up to 3 days. When ready to eat, warm in the microwave; then top with syrup and nuts.

PER SERVING *(3 ounces)*: Protein: 4g; Calories: 195; Fat: 10g; Carbohydrates: 27g; Fiber: 6g; Total sugar: 19g; Added sugar: 0g; Sodium: 4mg

FLOURLESS LOW-SUGAR PEANUT BUTTER BITES

5 Ingredients or Fewer

MAKES 8 // **PREP TIME**: 15 minutes, plus 20 minutes to chill // **COOK TIME**: 10 minutes

These soft, fluffy peanut butter bites melt in your mouth, are low in sugar, and contain no flour. You can dip them in milk or pair with 1 tablespoon of sugar-free ice cream. You can eat them warm right out of the oven or store them in a cookie jar for any time a craving strikes. But whatever you do, do not skip the 20 minutes of chill time—otherwise you may end up with a thin, flat cookie. Use a peanut butter with only peanuts and salt for ingredients, and skip any with added hydrogenated oils or sugar. Or try this recipe with sunflower seed butter.

1 large egg

⅓ cup creamy peanut butter

3 tablespoons packed light brown sugar

1 teaspoon vanilla extract

¼ teaspoon baking soda

1. Preheat the oven to 350°F. Line a small baking sheet with parchment paper or nonstick aluminum foil. Set aside.

2. In a small bowl, combine the egg, peanut butter, brown sugar, vanilla, and baking soda. Using a fork, mix well until you get a smooth consistency. Scoop the dough in 1-tablespoon portions onto the prepared baking sheet, spaced at least 2 inches apart. This should yield about 8 cookies. Using a fork or spoon, flatten each cookie slightly.

3. Place the baking sheet in the freezer for 20 minutes or longer before baking. (Warm dough will spread when baking, yielding a thinner and flatter cookie. Chilling will help the cookies keep their form.) You can also leave the dough in the freezer for a few days and bake the cookies at a later date.

4. Bake for 10 minutes.

5. Remove from the oven and let cool and harden on the baking sheet for about 10 minutes before enjoying.

STORAGE TIP: These bites will keep in a plastic zip-top bag or cookie jar at room temperature for 3 to 4 days. Cool the cookies completely before storing. Unbaked dough can be refrigerated in an airtight container for up to 5 days and baked as needed.

PER SERVING *(1 bite)*: Protein: 3g; Calories: 93; Fat: 6g; Carbohydrates: 8g; Fiber: 1g; Total sugar: 6g; Added sugar: 5g; Sodium: 50mg

RICOTTA-STUFFED STRAWBERRIES

SERVES 2 // **PREP TIME:** 10 minutes

5 Ingredients or Fewer
30 Minutes or Less
No Cook
One Pot

These strawberries are filled with light ricotta to create a deliciously healthy treat. This dessert is low in carbohydrates, low in sugar, and easy to make. It is a wonderful combination of flavors and textures and can be enjoyed after a meal or as a snack. Instead of sugar-free syrup, use stevia, maple syrup, or honey.

¼ cup part-skim ricotta

3 drops vanilla extract

3 drops sugar-free vanilla syrup (optional)

4 large fresh strawberries

1 tablespoon finely chopped toasted pecans

1. In a small bowl, combine the ricotta, vanilla, and syrup for extra sweetness (if using). Mix well.

2. Trim the bottom off each strawberry—just enough so it will stand up on its own. Then cut off the top and carve out the middle. Fill the strawberries with the sweetened ricotta mixture.

3. Sprinkle the berries with the pecans and enjoy.

COOKING TIP: Consider drizzling the filled berries with melted regular or sugar-free dark chocolate for added decadence. Sprinkle with any kind of nuts you prefer. And, if you don't want to fuss with carving each berry, dice them and top with the ricotta mixture and pecans.

PER SERVING *(2 stuffed strawberries)*: Protein: 4g; Calories: 78; Fat: 5g; Carbohydrates: 5g; Fiber: 1g; Total sugar: 2g; Added sugar: 0g; Sodium: 31mg

NO-BAKE CHOCOLATE-COCONUT BALLS

5 Ingredients or Fewer
30 Minutes or Less
No Cook
One Pot

MAKES 8 // **PREP TIME**: 10 minutes, plus up to 15 minutes to chill

I love making these chocolate balls. Just one is enough to satisfy your sweet tooth, and they don't require refrigeration (though they will last longer if kept in the refrigerator), so you can take them with you for an on-the-go snack. As a bonus, these no-bake balls are dairy-free, gluten-free, salt-free, and vegan, and you can make them organic by selecting only organic ingredients. Try this recipe with thick sugar-free syrup (the consistency of maple syrup), which can be found in the breakfast aisle, or with maple syrup.

¼ cup almond meal

¼ cup shredded unsweetened coconut flakes

2 tablespoons unsweetened cacao powder

2 tablespoons sugar-free breakfast syrup

1. In a medium bowl, combine the almond meal, coconut, cacao powder, and syrup. Using a fork or spoon, mix very well.

2. Scoop out ¾-tablespoon portions and roll each into a small ball. This should yield roughly 8 balls.

3. Enjoy immediately, or refrigerate for 10 to 15 minutes before serving.

COOKING TIP: For added protein, swap cacao powder for chocolate protein powder. Also, add chopped nuts, dates, or ground cinnamon for texture and flavor.

STORAGE TIP: Keep these balls in a plastic zip-top bag or airtight container for 3 to 5 days.

PER SERVING *(1 ball)*: Protein: 1g; Calories: 42; Fat: 4g; Carbohydrates: 3g; Fiber: 1g; Total sugar: <1g; Added sugar: 0g; Sodium: 9mg

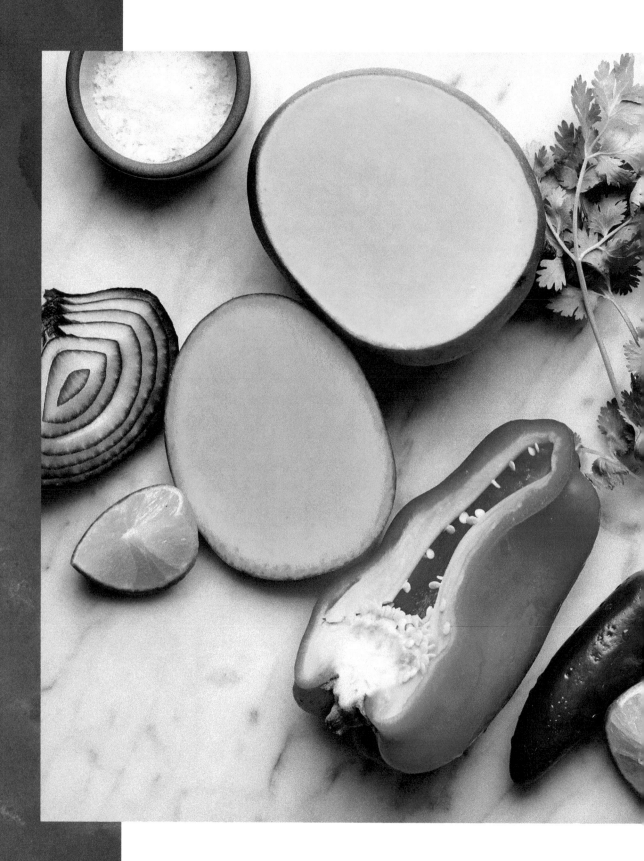

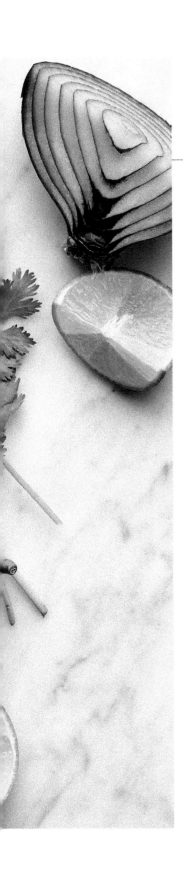

CHAPTER TWELVE

STAPLES

MANGO SALSA

MAKES 1 cup // **PREP TIME**: 20 minutes

5 Ingredients or Fewer
30 Minutes or Less
No Cook
One Pot

It's almost impossible to resist this sweet and spicy salsa, which adds an amazing burst of flavor to vegetarian meals, seafood, and even beef recipes. Full of antioxidants and fiber from the fruits, vegetables, and herbs, this colorful salsa can be prepared on a weekend and eaten over the next few days. If you prefer hot salsa, include the jalapeño.

1 ripe mango, peeled, pitted, and diced

½ red bell pepper, diced

¼ cup chopped red onion

2 tablespoons finely chopped fresh cilantro leaves

1 jalapeño pepper, seeded and finely diced (optional)

Juice of 1 lime (about 2 tablespoons)

Salt

1. In a small bowl, stir together the mango, red bell pepper, red onion, cilantro, and jalapeño (if using).

2. Drizzle with the lime juice. Taste and season with salt. Mix well.

COOKING TIP: This salsa tastes best if left to marinate for at least 10 minutes before eating. Refrigerate leftovers in an airtight container for up to 3 days.

PER SERVING *(2 tablespoons)*: Protein: 1g; Calories: 30; Fat: <1g; Carbohydrates: 7g; Fiber: 1g; Total sugar: 6g; Added sugar: 0g; Sodium: 1mg

SUNDRIED TOMATO PESTO

MAKES 1 cup // **PREP TIME:** 15 minutes, plus
10 minutes to cool

5 Ingredients or Fewer
30 Minutes or Less
No Cook

This is my favorite recipe in this book. Just one spoonful of this sweet, savory pesto can enhance any dish. Try it in a sandwich or wrap instead of mayonnaise. Add it to your salad, seafood, soup, or vegetarian meal. Spread it on crackers as a snack. Just be mindful: You should not consume more than 1 to 2 tablespoons per day. I use regular almonds in this recipe because they are the easiest nut to find; however, this pesto tastes even better made with toasted pine nuts or Marcona almonds. If you have it, include ½ cup of fresh basil instead of the dried basil.

1 cup dry-packed sun-dried tomatoes (not packed in oil)

¾ cup olive oil

⅓ cup unsalted dry-roasted almonds

3 garlic cloves, peeled

1 tablespoon dried basil

½ teaspoon red pepper flakes (optional)

¼ teaspoon salt, plus more as needed

¼ teaspoon freshly ground black pepper, plus more as needed

1. In a medium bowl, combine the sundried tomatoes with enough hot water to cover and let sit for 5 to 10 minutes, or until soft. Drain the liquid. Place the tomatoes in the refrigerator for about 10 minutes to cool.

2. In a blender or food processor, combine the cooled, soaked tomatoes, oil, almonds, garlic, basil, red pepper flakes (if using), salt, and black pepper. Process until the ingredients form a paste-like consistency. Taste and season with more salt and pepper, as needed.

STORAGE TIP: Refrigerate this pesto in an airtight container for 7 to 9 days, or freeze for up to 6 months. To freeze pesto, spoon single servings into an ice-cube tray and freeze for 2 hours. Remove the cubes—dipping the bottom of tray in hot water helps—and transfer them to a freezer-safe plastic zip-top bag. Keep frozen until needed.

PER SERVING *(1 tablespoon)*: Protein: 1g; Calories: 115; Fat: 12g; Carbohydrates: 3g; Fiber: 1g; Total sugar: 1g; Added sugar: 0g; Sodium: 41mg

PARMESAN CRISPS

MAKES 3 crisps // **PREP TIME:** 5 minutes // **COOK TIME:** 5 minutes

5 Ingredients or Fewer
30 Minutes or Less
One Pot

This recipe is probably the easiest one in the book: It has just one ingredient. These crisps are great paired with soups in place of crackers, broken over salads as a crunchy crouton replacement, or on their own as a snack. You can add variety with poppy seeds, sesame seeds, various spices, or dried onion or chives.

6 tablespoons shredded or freshly grated Parmesan cheese

1. Preheat the oven to 350°F. Line a baking sheet with nonstick aluminum foil.

2. Spoon the Parmesan cheese into three equal 2-tablespoon mounds, a few inches apart on the prepared baking sheet. Spread each mound into a 3-inch circle.

3. Bake for 5 minutes, or until the cheese is golden.

4. Let cool completely on the baking sheet until the cheese crisp hardens; then remove with a thin spatula.

STORAGE TIP: Store in an airtight container on the counter for up to 1 week.

PER SERVING *(1 crisp; ½ ounce)*: Protein: 5g; Calories: 55; Fat: 4g; Carbohydrates: 1g; Fiber: 0g; Total sugar: 1g; Added sugar: 0g; Sodium: 166mg

HERB QUINOA

MAKES 1¼ cups // **PREP TIME**: 5 minutes // **COOK TIME**: 15 minutes

5 Ingredients or Fewer
30 Minutes or Less
One Pot

This fast, simple quinoa is one of my go-to staples for a quick, healthy side. It is easy to make, requires little prep time, and tastes great when reheated—plus, quinoa is high in protein and fiber. To change up the recipe and add extra flavor, use a flavored olive oil or combine it with basil pesto or Sundried Tomato Pesto (page 169). Parsley can be swapped for basil or cilantro. You can also use low-sodium broth instead of water to cook the quinoa.

½ cup raw quinoa, rinsed well

1 cup water

Salt

2 tablespoons finely chopped fresh parsley

2 teaspoons olive oil

Garlic powder, for seasoning

1. In a medium pot over high heat, combine the quinoa and water. Season with salt to taste and bring to a boil. Cover the pot and reduce the heat to low. Simmer for about 15 minutes until all the water is absorbed. When done, the quinoa should look soft and translucent, and a germ curl will be visible along the outside edge of the grain.

2. Stir in the parsley and oil and season with garlic powder to taste.

COOKING TIP: If you have time, sauté fresh garlic, chopped onion, and chopped carrot in the olive oil and add them to the quinoa for added flavor.

STORAGE TIP: Refrigerate leftover quinoa in an airtight container for up to 3 days, or freeze for up to 6 months.

PER SERVING (¼ cup): Protein: 2g; Calories: 79; Fat: 3g; Carbohydrates: 11g; Fiber: 1g; Total sugar: 1g; Added sugar: 0g; Sodium: 2mg

GARLIC CAULIFLOWER AND POTATO MASH

5 Ingredients or Fewer

MAKES 2 cups // **PREP TIME**: 10 minutes // **COOK TIME**: 25 minutes

This easy carbohydrate option pairs well with vegetarian dishes, chicken, fish, and meat. It can be consumed on the soft diet as well. I like it better with the scallions. If you don't have fresh garlic, use bottled minced garlic or 1 teaspoon of garlic powder.

2 russet potatoes, halved and peeled

2 large garlic cloves, minced

2 cups chopped cauliflower florets

3 tablespoons nonfat milk

2 tablespoons olive oil

Salt

Freshly ground black pepper

Chopped scallion or fresh chives, for garnish (optional)

1. In a medium pot, combine the potatoes, garlic, and enough cold water to cover the potatoes by 2 to 3 inches. Bring to a boil over high heat and cook for about 15 minutes until the potatoes are about half cooked.

2. Add the cauliflower and more water if needed and cook for about 10 more minutes, or until the potatoes and cauliflower are soft. Drain.

3. Place the potatoes and cauliflower in a medium bowl. Add the milk and oil and season with salt and pepper to taste. Using a potato masher or fork, mash the vegetables until well combined. Garnish with scallion (if using) when serving and enjoy.

COOKING TIP: For extra flavor, add sautéed garlic or onion just before you mash the potatoes and cauliflower.

STORAGE TIP: Refrigerate in an airtight container for up to 4 days, or freeze for up to 3 months. Reheat when ready to use.

PER SERVING (½ cup): Protein: 4g; Calories: 164; Fat: 7g; Carbohydrates: 23g; Fiber: 3g; Total sugar: 2g; Added sugar: 0g; Sodium: 27mg

MEASUREMENT CONVERSIONS

VOLUME EQUIVALENTS	U.S. STANDARD	U.S. STANDARD (OUNCES)	METRIC (APPROXIMATE)
LIQUID	2 tablespoons	1 fl. oz.	30 mL
	¼ cup	2 fl. oz.	60 mL
	½ cup	4 fl. oz.	120 mL
	1 cup	8 fl. oz.	240 mL
	1½ cups	12 fl. oz.	355 mL
	2 cups or 1 pint	16 fl. oz.	475 mL
	4 cups or 1 quart	32 fl. oz.	1 L
	1 gallon	128 fl. oz.	4 L
DRY	⅛ teaspoon	–	0.5 mL
	¼ teaspoon	–	1 mL
	½ teaspoon	–	2 mL
	¾ teaspoon	–	4 mL
	1 teaspoon	–	5 mL
	1 tablespoon	–	15 mL
	¼ cup	–	59 mL
	⅓ cup	–	79 mL
	½ cup	–	118 mL
	⅔ cup	–	156 mL
	¾ cup	–	177 mL
	1 cup	–	235 mL
	2 cups or 1 pint	–	475 mL
	3 cups	–	700 mL
	4 cups or 1 quart	–	1 L
	½ gallon	–	2 L
	1 gallon	–	4 L

OVEN TEMPERATURES

FAHRENHEIT	CELSIUS (APPROXIMATE)
250°F	120°C
300°F	150°C
325°F	165°C
350°F	180°C
375°F	190°C
400°F	200°C
425°F	220°C
450°F	230°C

WEIGHT EQUIVALENTS

U.S. STANDARD	METRIC (APPROXIMATE)
½ ounce	15 g
1 ounce	30 g
2 ounces	60 g
4 ounces	115 g
8 ounces	225 g
12 ounces	340 g
16 ounces or 1 pound	455 g

RESOURCES

Websites

ASMBS.org
Visit the website of the American Society for Metabolic and Bariatric Surgery for more information about surgery, surgeons in your area, and diet after surgery.

EatRight.org
This website from the Academy of Nutrition and Dietetics provides healthy eating ideas, recipes, weight-loss tips, reputable nutrition information, and more.

ObesityHelp.com
This website includes helpful information about bariatric surgery and support for bariatric patients after surgery, including healthy recipes, tips for weight loss and maintaining weight loss, and more.

Books

Eat to Beat Disease: The New Science of How Your Body Can Heal Itself, **William W. Li, MD**
I suggest reading this book six or more months after surgery. It explains the foods that you should eat to heal the body and prevent chronic diseases.

Intuitive Eating: An Anti-Diet Revolutionary Approach, **4th ed., Evelyn Tribole, MS, RDN, and Elyse Resch, MS, RDN**
This book will help you overcome the diet mindset and find pleasure in eating as well as explain reasons for hunger and cravings and what may cause overeating. It will also improve your relationship with food and help you avoid distracted eating.

The Psychology of Overeating: Food and the Culture of Consumerism, **Kima Cargill**
This book explains the reasons people overeat and how the food industry uses psychology to trick consumers into buying more food.

Supplements

As mentioned earlier in this book, supplementation is crucial after VSG. Following are the bariatric supplements currently available on the market. As always, please discuss your best option, based on your preferences, lifestyle, and budget, with your surgeon. I recommend contacting the companies and requesting a variety of samples to try before determining which option is best.

Bariatric Advantage, BariatricAdvantage.com
One of the first companies to make supplements for VSG patients, Bariatric Advantage has a large variety of vitamin and mineral supplements as well as protein shakes and powders.

Bariatric Fusion, BariatricFusion.com
Here you'll find a great variety of supplements, protein drinks, and bars.

BariMelts, BariMelts.com
This option is a "chewable" vitamin tablet that melts in your mouth. It is convenient for the first weeks after surgery and tastes good.

Celebrate Nutritional Supplements, CelebrateVitamins.com
Celebrate offers a large assortment of supplements, protein drinks, snacks, and treats. It can be one-stop shop for all your supplements.

Fit for Me, FitForMe.com
Based in Europe, this company offers affordable multivitamins for weight-loss surgery patients tailored to their individual post-op needs.

ProCare Health, ProCareNow.com
This company offers a variety of chewable capsules, meal-replacement shakes, and even a dark chocolate calcium supplement.

Unjury, Unjury.com
Founded by a dietitian and her husband, this company offers supplements, bars, ready-to-go drinks, and one of the best-quality unflavored protein powders on the market.

INDEX

ACKNOWLEDGMENTS

I would like to thank...

My mom and dad, Nina and Alexander, who taught me how to cook and make something from nothing as soon as I was able to hold a spoon. My American family, Terri and Dennis, who taught me about global cuisines by taking me to restaurants in many countries and introducing me to chefs from different parts of the world.

The first bariatric surgeon I worked with, Dr. Bobby Bhasker-Rao, in Southern California, who gave me my first job as a Registered Dietitian and supported me.

Jeanne Blankenship, MS, RDN, who was my first mentor in bariatric nutrition and gave me the guidance needed to start my career.

All the dietitians I have had the pleasure of working with, who shared their knowledge and expertise and who help patients eat healthier and change their lifestyle. I am especially thankful for my coworkers, known as "The Real Dietitians of Orange County," who have been supportive of my career and took the time to test my recipes.

Kathy Pham, RDN, who has always encouraged my efforts, and has been a true role model in the field of nutrition and dietetics.

My dear friend Yasi Ansari, MS, RDN, who always supported and encouraged me to keep going, and Viktoria Waite, MS, RDN, my friend and assistant, who helps me with my work, projects, and ideas.

Ashley Popp and Callisto Media, who gave me the opportunity to create this book. And tremendous thanks to my editor, Rachelle Cihonski, who gave me the freedom to write and was open to my ideas.

You have all been part of my journey, and I cannot thank you enough.

ABOUT THE AUTHOR

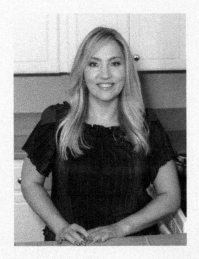

Marina Savelyeva, RD, CNSC, has been a registered dietitian for more than 15 years. She has worked in hospitals, collaborated with bariatric and gastrointestinal surgeons, and helped numerous clients via her private practice. Nutrition and food science have always been passions of hers. Savelyeva continues to stay up-to-date with the latest research and incorporates evidenced-based practices into her work with clients. She enjoys cooking and loves to travel. Her passion is to help people live healthy lives by adopting practices that are easy to follow! She enjoys seeing her patients succeed in their health journeys.

Printed in the USA
CPSIA information can be obtained
at www.ICGtesting.com
LVHW061538191123
763966LV00001B/6